Current Management of Hip Fracture

Current Management of Hip Fracture

Editor

Carsten Schoeneberg

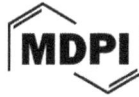

Basel • Beijing • Wuhan • Barcelona • Belgrade • Novi Sad • Cluj • Manchester

Editor
Carsten Schoeneberg
Department of Orthopedic
and Emergency Surgery
Alfried Krupp Hospital
Essen, Germany

Editorial Office
MDPI
St. Alban-Anlage 66
4052 Basel, Switzerland

This is a reprint of articles from the Special Issue published online in the open access journal *Medicina* (ISSN 1648-9144) (available at: https://www.mdpi.com/journal/medicina/special_issues/Hip_Orthogeriatric).

For citation purposes, cite each article independently as indicated on the article page online and as indicated below:

Lastname, A.A.; Lastname, B.B. Article Title. *Journal Name* **Year**, *Volume Number*, Page Range.

ISBN 978-3-7258-0051-3 (Hbk)
ISBN 978-3-7258-0052-0 (PDF)
doi.org/10.3390/books978-3-7258-0052-0

© 2024 by the authors. Articles in this book are Open Access and distributed under the Creative Commons Attribution (CC BY) license. The book as a whole is distributed by MDPI under the terms and conditions of the Creative Commons Attribution-NonCommercial-NoDerivs (CC BY-NC-ND) license.

Contents

Preface vii

Carsten Schoeneberg
Current Management of Hip Fracture
Reprinted from: *Medicina* **2023**, *59*, 26, doi:10.3390/medicina59010026 1

Giuseppe Di Martino, Pamela Di Giovanni, Fabrizio Cedrone, Michela D'Addezio, Francesca Meo, Piera Scampoli, et al.
Development and Validation of a New Tool in Predicting In-Hospital Mortality for Hip-Fractured Patients: The PRIMOF Score
Reprinted from: *Medicina* **2022**, *58*, 1082, doi:10.3390/medicina58081082 5

Christopher Bliemel, Katherine Rascher, Ludwig Oberkircher, Torsten Schlosshauer, Carsten Schoeneberg, Matthias Knobe, et al.
Surgical Management and Outcomes Following Pathologic Hip Fracture—Results from a Propensity Matching Analysis of the Registry for Geriatric Trauma of the German Trauma Society
Reprinted from: *Medicina* **2022**, *58*, 871, doi:10.3390/medicina58070871 12

Riccardo Giorgino, Erfan Soroush, Sajjad Soroush, Sara Malakouti, Haniyeh Salari, Valeria Vismara, et al.
COVID-19 Elderly Patients Treated for Proximal Femoral Fractures during the Second Wave of Pandemic in Italy and Iran: A Comparison between Two Countries
Reprinted from: *Medicina* **2022**, *58*, 781, doi:10.3390/medicina58060781 25

Marcel Niemann, Karl F. Braun, Sufian S. Ahmad, Ulrich Stöckle, Sven Märdian and Frank Graef
Comparing Perioperative Outcome Measures of the Dynamic Hip Screw and the Femoral Neck System
Reprinted from: *Medicina* **2022**, *58*, 352, doi:10.3390/medicina58030352 32

Simon Hackl, Christian von Rüden, Ferdinand Weisemann, Isabella Klöpfer-Krämer, Fabian M. Stuby and Florian Högel
Internal Fixation of Garden Type III Femoral Neck Fractures with Sliding Hip Screw and Anti-Rotation Screw: Does Increased Valgus Improve Healing?
Reprinted from: *Medicina* **2022**, *58*, 1573, doi:10.3390/medicina58111573 42

Emanuel Kuner, Jens Gütler, Dimitri E. Delagrammaticas, Bryan J. M. van de Wall, Matthias Knobe, Frank J. P. Beeres, et al.
High Percentage of Complications and Re-Operations Following Dynamic Locking Plate Fixation with the Targon® FN for Intracapsular Proximal Femoral Fractures: An Analysis of Risk Factors
Reprinted from: *Medicina* **2022**, *58*, 1812, doi:10.3390/medicina58121812 54

Ulf Bökeler, Alissa Bühler, Daphne Eschbach, Christoph Ilies, Ulrich Liener and Tom Knauf
The Influence of a Modified 3rd Generation Cementation Technique and Vaccum Mixing of Bone Cement on the Bone Cement Implantation Syndrome (BCIS) in Geriatric Patients with Cemented Hemiarthroplasty for Femoral Neck Fractures
Reprinted from: *Medicina* **2022**, *58*, 1587, doi:10.3390/medicina58111587 67

Torsten Pastor, Ivan Zderic, Clemens Schopper, Pascal C. Haefeli, Philipp Kastner, Firas Souleiman, et al.
Impact of Anterior Malposition and Bone Cement Augmentation on the Fixation Strength of Cephalic Intramedullary Nail Head Elements
Reprinted from: *Medicina* **2022**, *58*, 1636, doi:10.3390/medicina58111636 77

Yu-Pin Chen, Wei-Chun Chang, Tsai-Wei Wen, Pei-Chun Chien, Shu-Wei Huang and Yi-Jie Kuo
Multipronged Programmatic Strategy for Preventing Secondary Fracture and Facilitating Functional Recovery in Older Patients after Hip Fractures: Our Experience in Taipei Municipal Wanfang Hospital
Reprinted from: *Medicina* **2022**, *58*, 875, doi:10.3390/medicina58070875 89

Moritz Kraus, Carl Neuerburg, Nicole Thomasser, Ulla Cordula Stumpf, Matthias Blaschke, Werner Plötz, et al.
Reduced Awareness for Osteoporosis in Hip Fracture Patients Compared to Elderly Patients Undergoing Elective Hip Replacement
Reprinted from: *Medicina* **2022**, *58*, 1564, doi:10.3390/medicina58111564 100

Nicola Maffulli and Rocco Aicale
Proximal Femoral Fractures in the Elderly: A Few Things to Know, and Some to Forget
Reprinted from: *Medicina* **2022**, *58*, 1314, doi:10.3390/medicina58101314 111

Preface

Due to demographic changes and aging populations, the incidence of hip fracture, as a typical fragility fracture, is increasing worldwide. Because of the patients' age, existing comorbidities, reduced daily life activities, poor bone quality, and preexisting implants, the treatment of hip fractures can be challenging. Therefore, proximal femur fractures are often life-changing events in older adults and are associated with a high mortality rate: up to 35% after 1 year. Moreover, these fractures are associated with decreased walking ability, decreased quality of life, and the loss of independence. Moreover, hip fractures are associated with high socioeconomic costs, due to surgical complications, reduced coping capacities, and high institutionalization rates.

These dramatic consequences have led to the development of optimized implants and the establishment of orthogeriatric co-management. This concept indicates multi-professional and interdisciplinary cooperation between surgeons and geriatric specialists. The advantages of such a cooperation are evident from the reduction in mortality and complications. In addition, special national guidelines have been established to provide the best care of hip fracture patients.

Moreover, special geriatric hip fracture registries have been established in different countries. These registries enable the analysis of big data and have the potential to improve the treatment of geriatric hip fracture patients.

However, in most countries worldwide, there is a large supply gap in the prevention of secondary fractures following fragility fractures. For example, in the United States, the prevalence of pre- and post-fracture anti-osteoporotic medication is under 25%. Similar results are reported from China, Italy, Germany, and other countries.

The body of literature concerning hip fracture has risen exponentially in the past few years. Nevertheless, due to the divergence of the reported results, several questions remain unanswered, like what the predictors are for worse outcomes, what easy-to-use predictor scores are available, what the best time-to-surgery is, what the best implant for the individual patient is, whether a cement augmentation should be performed, what the best concept of orthogeriatric co-management is, and much more.

The purpose of this Special Issue is to discuss the evidence surrounding the current management of hip fractures. Therefore, the scope is not only tailored to surgical strategies and the choice of implant, but should also focus on the whole process of treating patients suffering a hip fracture. This includes epidemiology, process optimization, orthogeriatric co-management concepts, geriatric fracture centers, and the secondary prevention of fractures. Moreover, analyses of the socioeconomic consequences are also of interest.

Carsten Schoeneberg
Editor

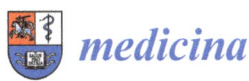

Editorial

Current Management of Hip Fracture

Carsten Schoeneberg

Department of Orthopedic and Emergency Surgery, Alfried Krupp Hospital, 45276 Essen, Germany; carsten.schoeneberg@krupp-krankenhaus.de

Keywords: hip fracture; Geriatric Trauma; orthogeriatric co-management; proximal femur fracture; Geriatric Trauma registry

This Special Issue, entitled "Current Management of Hip Fracture", ran in the *Medicina* journal of MDPI's "Surgery" section, reports the findings of international studies regarding different aspects in the treatment of patients suffering a proximal femur fracture. Therefore, the results of these studies are not only tailored to surgical strategies and the choice of implant, but also focus on the whole process of treating hip fracture patients. This Special Issue presents the entire treatment process. Starting with a pre-surgery risk stratification, we highlight the results of studies into different newer implants and strategies for the surgical treatment of hip fractures, as well as the impact of patient-associated factors, like malnutrition and anticoagulation, on outcomes after hip fractures are diagnosed. Two studies focus on the prevention of secondary fractures and the often-underlying osteoporosis. This issue also includes a biomechanical study which presents the impact of malposition and bone cement augmentation on fixation strength. Finally, a review of the current literature attempts to summarize the current knowledge in the treatment of hip fractures.

A total of 13 published articles demonstrate the importance of this issue and its interest to the scientific society.

Di Martino et al. present a new score, called the PRIMOF Score, to predict in-hospital mortality rates for hip fracture patients. In this retrospective study, they include over 23,000 patients, aged over 40 years, from the Abruzzo region in Italy. They split the cohort into two equal groups—the training sample and the validation sample. The final score ranges from 0 to 27 and is divided into four risk categories. This simple score, which is based on patient characteristics and clinical comorbidities, can stratify the risk of in-hospital mortality in hip fracture patients [1].

Aigner et al. analyze the effect of direct anticoagulants on the treatment of geriatric patients with a hip fracture. They conduct a registry-based analysis of 15,099 patients from the German Registry for Geriatric Trauma (ATR-DGU). They find that the time-to-surgery is prolonged in patients receiving anticoagulation drugs. However, no significant differences regarding complications, type of anesthesia and mortality are observed. They conclude that "even in the absence of widely available antidotes, the safe management of geriatric patients under DOACs with proximal femur fractures is possible" [2].

Another study from the ATR-DGU analyzes the surgical management and outcomes of pathologic hip fractures. Bliemel et al. report no differences between pathologic and osteoporotic fractures during initial hospital treatment in regard of mortality, reoperation rate and walking ability. However, in the follow-up period of 120 days, the mortality rate in pathologic hip fractures is found to be three times higher. Further, they find that pathologic per- and subtrochanteric fractures are more frequently treated by arthroplasty compared to osteoporotic fractures [3].

Pass et al. analyze the influence of malnutrition on the outcome of geriatric hip fractures, in addition to the impact of hypalbuminemia and body mass index. They conclude

Citation: Schoeneberg, C. Current Management of Hip Fracture. *Medicina* **2023**, *59*, 26. https://doi.org/10.3390/medicina59010026

Received: 12 December 2022
Revised: 16 December 2022
Accepted: 21 December 2022
Published: 23 December 2022

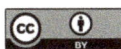

Copyright: © 2022 by the author. Licensee MDPI, Basel, Switzerland. This article is an open access article distributed under the terms and conditions of the Creative Commons Attribution (CC BY) license (https://creativecommons.org/licenses/by/4.0/).

that "Hypoalbuminemia might be an indicator for more vulnerable patients with a compromised hemoglobin level, prothrombin time, and ASA grade. Therefore, it is also associated with higher mortality rate and postoperative complications. However, hypoalbuminemia was not an independent predictor for mortality or postoperative complications, but low albumin values were associated with a higher CCI and ASA grade than in patients with a BMI lower than 20 kg/m^2" [4].

Giorgino et al. compare the treatment of COVID-19-positive patients in Italy and Iran suffering from proximal femur fractures in terms of characteristics, comorbidities, outcomes and complications. They find that the Italian patients are older, receive more frequent transfusions of blood during their hospital stays, and that their hospital stays are longer [5].

Niemann et al. conduct a retrospective single-center study to compare the dynamic hip screw and the femoral neck system, a recently introduced system for the internal fixation of femoral neck fractures. There is no difference in fracture complexity between both groups. They find a nearly 50% reduction in operating time and dose area product with X-Rays in the femoral neck system group. These results significantly differ, meaning that the surgical treatment using the femoral neck system results in a shorter operating time and less fluoroscopy time [6].

Hackl et al., in a retrospective single-center study, analyze the differences between valgus and anatomical reposition in Garden type III femoral neck fractures, treated with a sliding hip screw and anti-rotation screw. They exclusively include patients younger than 70 years of age. They report a significantly lower failure rate and shorter healing time in the anatomical reposition group [7].

In their retrospective single-center study, Kuner et al. analyze the outcome of intracapsular proximal femur fractures treated with the Targon® FN, a dynamic locking plate fixation. They include 72 cases, in which 34 patients (47.2%) have experienced one or more complications, the most common of these being a mechanical irritation of the iliotibial band. Moreover, 46 re-operations were required. They conclude that "the Targon-FN system resulted in a high rate of post-operative complication and re-operation. Statistical analysis revealed patient age, fracture displacement, time to postoperative full weight bearing were risk factors for re-operation" [8].

One study, entitled "The influence of a Modified 3rd Generation Cementation Technique and Vacuum Mixing of Bone Cement on the Bone Cement Implantation Syndrome (BCIS) in Geriatric Patients with Cemented Hemiarthroplasty for Femoral Neck Fractures", is published by Bökeler et al. They compare 2nd and 3rd generation cementing techniques. The incidence and early mortality are found to be significantly higher in the 2nd generation cementing technique group. Therefore, the authors decide to use a 3rd generation cementing technique [9].

A biomechanical analysis from the AO Research Institute Davos is published by Pastor et al. They compare the differences between the helical blade and the screw as head elements of the Trochanteric Femoral Nail Advanced System, either in center–center position or anterior off-center position, and the effect of bone cement augmentation. They conclude that "From a biomechanical perspective, proper centre–centre implant positioning in the femoral head is of utmost importance. In cases when this is not achievable in a clinical setting, a helical blade is more forgiving in the less ideal (anterior) position when compared to a screw, the latter revealing unacceptable low resistance to femoral head rotation and early failure. Cement augmentation of both off-centre implanted helical blade and screw head elements increases their resistance against failure; however, this effect might be redundant for helical blades and is highly unpredictable for screws" [10].

Chen et al. report the effectiveness of a fracture liaison service after 1 year of implementation at a Taipei Municipal hospital. The implementation of a fracture liaison service increases the osteoporotic treatment after hip fracture from 22.8% to 72.3% and decreases the re-fracture rate from 11.8% to 4.9%. The one-year mortality rate decreases from 17.9% to 11.8%. However, this does not reach statistical significance. They conclude that a fracture liaison service has the potential to improve the outcomes and care quality after hip fracture surgery [11].

Kraus et al. compare the awareness for osteoporosis in hip fracture patients to elderly patients undergoing elective hip arthroplasty. Although the FRAX® Score is significantly different between these two groups, they determine that the fracture group has a considerably greater risk for another osteoporotic fracture and that the patients of this group show a reduced awareness of osteoporosis. Moreover, the willingness to participate in other screening programs, like colonoscopy and check-ups, is higher in both groups. The authors discuss that the reduced awareness of osteoporosis might be one factor in the low rate of osteoporotic treatment in elderly patients. They conclude that the "implementation of a screening and care program for osteoporosis such as Fracture Liaison Services (FLS) may improve patient awareness of this condition, especially among fracture patients" [12].

In a review entitled "Proximal Femoral Fractures in the Elderly: A Few Things to Know, and Some to Forget", Maffulli and Aicale present the current literature in relation to the peri-operative, the operative, and the postoperative treatment. They define the management of hip fracture patients as a coordinated multidisciplinary approach, with early surgery, pain treatment, balanced fluid therapy, and prevention of delirium as fundamental in the treatment. The operative treatments for inter- or subtrochanteric fractures are intramedullary nailing or dynamic hip screw, and in case of neck fractures, total hip replacement or hemiarthroplasty. Early mobilization and a geriatric multidisciplinary care could be beneficial for patients with hip fracture. Because of the multifactorial reasons for hip fractures and demanding challenges, the authors concluded, that the "Management cannot be limited only to the operating theatre. Given the increase in the burden of disease, the true challenge is in prevention and in developing strategies to improve the quality of life for this group of patients" [13].

In summary, this Special Issue presents a number of studies covering the whole treatment process of hip fracture patients. A novel pre-operative risk score to estimate in-hospital mortality is presented. Several studies analyzed the outcome of modern implants and intra-operative modifications to reach a good surgical care of hip fractures. The coherence and possible optimization of post-operative osteoporotic care are presented. Finally, a review of the current literature presents the latest standards of peri-operative, operative, and postoperative treatment. Therefore, this Special Issue presents a detailed overview of the "Current Management of Hip Fracture".

Funding: This research received no external funding.

Institutional Review Board Statement: Not applicable.

Informed Consent Statement: Not applicable.

Data Availability Statement: Not applicable.

Conflicts of Interest: The author declare no conflict of interest.

References

1. Di Martino, G.; Di Giovanni, P.; Cedrone, F.; D'Addezio, M.; Meo, F.; Scampoli, P.; Romano, F.; Staniscia, T. Development and Validation of a New Tool in Predicting In-Hospital Mortality for Hip-Fractured Patients: The PRIMOF Score. *Medicina* **2022**, *58*, 1082. [CrossRef]
2. Aigner, R.; Buecking, B.; Hack, J.; Schwenzfeur, R.; Eschbach, D.; Einheuser, J.; Schoeneberg, C.; Pass, B.; Ruchholtz, S.; Knauf, T.; et al. Effect of Direct Oral Anticoagulants on Treatment of Geriatric Hip Fracture Patients: An Analysis of 15,099 Patients of the AltersTraumaRegister DGU®. *Medicina* **2022**, *58*, 379. [CrossRef]
3. Bliemel, C.; Rascher, K.; Oberkircher, L.; Schlosshauer, T.; Schoeneberg, C.; Knobe, M.; Pass, B.; Ruchholtz, S.; Klasan, A.; on behalf of the AltersTraumaRegister DGU. Surgical Management and Outcomes following Pathologic Hip Fracture—Results from a Propensity Matching Analysis of the Registry for Geriatric Trauma of the German Trauma Society. *Medicina* **2022**, *58*, 871. [CrossRef] [PubMed]
4. Pass, B.; Malek, F.; Rommelmann, M.; Aigner, R.; Knauf, T.; Eschbach, D.; Hussmann, B.; Maslaris, A.; Lendemans, S.; Schoeneberg, C. The Influence of Malnutrition Measured by Hypalbuminemia and Body Mass Index on the Outcome of Geriatric Patients with a Fracture of the Proximal Femur. *Medicina* **2022**, *58*, 1610. [CrossRef] [PubMed]

5. Giorgino, R.; Soroush, E.; Soroush, S.; Malakouti, S.; Salari, H.; Vismara, V.; Migliorini, F.; Accetta, R.; Mangiavini, L. COVID-19 Elderly Patients Treated for Proximal Femoral Fractures during the Second Wave of Pandemic in Italy and Iran: A Comparison between Two Countries. *Medicina* **2022**, *58*, 781. [CrossRef] [PubMed]
6. Niemann, M.; Braun, K.F.; Ahmad, S.S.; Stöckle, U.; Märdian, S.; Graef, F. Comparing Perioperative Outcome Measures of the Dynamic Hip Screw and the Femoral Neck System. *Medicina* **2022**, *58*, 352. [CrossRef] [PubMed]
7. Hackl, S.; von Rüden, C.; Weisemann, F.; Klöpfer-Krämer, I.; Stuby, F.M.; Högel, F. Internal Fixation of Garden Type III Femoral Neck Fractures with Sliding Hip Screw and Anti-Rotation Screw: Does Increased Valgus Improve Healing? *Medicina* **2022**, *58*, 1573. [CrossRef] [PubMed]
8. Kuner, E.; Gütler, J.; Delagrammaticas, D.E.; van de Wall, B.J.M.; Knobe, M.; Beeres, F.J.P.; Babst, R.; Link, B.-C. High Percentage of Complications and Re-Operations Following Dynamic Locking Plate Fixation with the Targon® FN for Intracapsular Proximal Femoral Fractures: An Analysis of Risk Factors. *Medicina* **2022**, *58*, 1812. [CrossRef]
9. Bökeler, U.; Bühler, A.; Eschbach, D.; Ilies, C.; Liener, U.; Knauf, T. The Influence of a Modified 3rd Generation Cementation Technique and Vaccum Mixing of Bone Cement on the Bone Cement Implantation Syndrome (BCIS) in Geriatric Patients with Cemented Hemiarthroplasty for Femoral Neck Fractures. *Medicina* **2022**, *58*, 1587. [CrossRef] [PubMed]
10. Pastor, T.; Zderic, I.; Schopper, C.; Haefeli, P.C.; Kastner, P.; Souleiman, F.; Gueorguiev, B.; Knobe, M. Impact of Anterior Malposition and Bone Cement Augmentation on the Fixation Strength of Cephalic Intramedullary Nail Head Elements. *Medicina* **2022**, *58*, 1636. [CrossRef] [PubMed]
11. Chen, Y.-P.; Chang, W.-C.; Wen, T.-W.; Chien, P.-C.; Huang, S.-W.; Kuo, Y.-J. Multipronged Programmatic Strategy for Preventing Secondary Fracture and Facilitating Functional Recovery in Older Patients after Hip Fractures: Our Experience in Taipei Municipal Wanfang Hospital. *Medicina* **2022**, *58*, 875. [CrossRef] [PubMed]
12. Kraus, M.; Neuerburg, C.; Thomasser, N.; Stumpf, U.C.; Blaschke, M.; Plötz, W.; Saller, M.M.; Böcker, W.; Keppler, A.M. Reduced Awareness for Osteoporosis in Hip Fracture Patients Compared to Elderly Patients Undergoing Elective Hip Replacement. *Medicina* **2022**, *58*, 1564. [CrossRef] [PubMed]
13. Maffulli, N.; Aicale, R. Proximal Femoral Fractures in the Elderly: A Few Things to Know, and Some to Forget. *Medicina* **2022**, *58*, 1314. [CrossRef] [PubMed]

Disclaimer/Publisher's Note: The statements, opinions and data contained in all publications are solely those of the individual author(s) and contributor(s) and not of MDPI and/or the editor(s). MDPI and/or the editor(s) disclaim responsibility for any injury to people or property resulting from any ideas, methods, instructions or products referred to in the content.

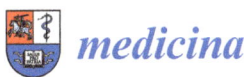

Article

Development and Validation of a New Tool in Predicting In-Hospital Mortality for Hip-Fractured Patients: The PRIMOF Score

Giuseppe Di Martino [1,2,*], Pamela Di Giovanni [3], Fabrizio Cedrone [2], Michela D'Addezio [4], Francesca Meo [4], Piera Scampoli [5], Ferdinando Romano [6] and Tommaso Staniscia [1]

1. Department of Medicine and Ageing Sciences, "G. d'Annunzio" University of Chieti-Pescara, 66100 Chieti, Italy
2. Unit of Hygiene, Epidemiology and Public Health, Local Health Authority of Pescara, 65100 Pescara, Italy
3. Department of Pharmacy, "G. d'Annunzio" University of Chieti-Pescara, 66100 Chieti, Italy
4. School of Hygiene and Preventive Medicine, "G. d'Annunzio" University of Chieti-Pescara, 66100 Chieti, Italy
5. Unit of Hygiene, Epidemiology and Public Health, Local Health Authority of Lanciano-Vasto-Chieti, 66100 Chieti, Italy
6. Department of Infectious Diseases and Public Health, "La Sapienza" University of Rome, 00185 Rome, Italy
* Correspondence: giuseppe.dimartino@unich.it; Tel.: +39-0871-355-4118

Abstract: *Background and Objectives*: The improved life expectancy was associated to the increased in the incidence of hip fractures among elderly people. Subjects suffering hip fractures frequently show concomitant conditions causing prolonged lengths of stay and higher in-hospital mortality. The knowledge of factors associated to in-hospital mortality or adverse events can help healthcare providers improve patients' outcomes and management. The aim of this study was to develop a score to predict in-hospital mortality among hip fractured patients. *Materials and Methods*: Cases were selected from hospital admissions that occurred during the period 2006–2015 in Abruzzo region, Italy. The study population was split into two random samples in order to evaluate the accuracy of prediction models. A multivariate logistic regression was performed in order to identify factors associated to in-hospital mortality. All diagnoses significantly associated to in-hospital mortality were included in the final model. *Results*: The PRIMOF ranged between 0 and 27 and was divided into four risk categories to allow the score interpretation. An increase in odds ratio values with the increase in PRIMOF score was reported in both study groups. *Conclusions*: This study showed that a simple score based on the patient' clinical comorbidities was able to stratify the risk of hip-fractured patients in terms of in-hospital mortality.

Keywords: hip fracture; mortality; prediction score; HDR; Italy

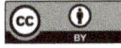

1. Introduction

The improved life expectancy was associated to the increase in the incidence of hip fractures among elderly people. Patients suffering hip fractures frequently show concomitant conditions causing prolonged lengths of stay and higher in-hospital mortality [1]. Hence, hip fractures in the geriatric population constitute a significant global public health issue [2,3]. The knowledge of factors associated to in-hospital mortality or adverse events can help healthcare providers improve patients' outcomes and management [4]. In the scientific literature, various scoring tools have been developed to predict in-hospital mortality, though it is uncertain which of these is the most useful for patients with hip fractures. In particular, most of them—i.e., the Charlson Comorbidity Index [5] or POSSUM score [6]—have been adapted for surgical risk stratification, but none of them were specifically developed for hip-fractured patients. Some tools have been developed for hip-fractured patients [7], but they are frequently not easy to use. The ideal risk scoring should be simple, user-friendly, reproducible, and available to all patients, as reported by Jones et al. [8]. To this extent, the aim of this study was the development and validation of the "PRedict In-hospital MOrtality of hip Fractured" (PRIMOF) score, a predictive model derived from hospital discharge records. The secondary aim was to compare it with the Charlson Comorbidity Index (CCI), one of the most common tools used in risk stratification, in terms of discrimination.

2. Materials and Methods

2.1. Data Source

The study was conducted in Abruzzo, a Southern Italian region [9]. Patients were chosen from the hospital discharge record (HDR) referred to admissions that occurred during years 2006–2015. HDR included information about the demographic characteristics of each patient, a Diagnosis Related Group code (DRG) used to classify the hospitalization, and up to six possible diagnoses (one principal diagnosis and five possible comorbidities) and up to six possible procedures performed during the hospital stay, coded according to the International Classification of Disease, 9th Revision, Clinical Modification (ICD-9-CM).

2.2. Inclusion Criteria

All patients aged over 40 years admitted in the Abruzzo region for HF were included in the study. Only admissions reporting the codes from 820.0 to 820.9 (hip fracture) in the HDR as their diagnosis were included in the analysis. Additionally, the most frequent comorbidities reporting a prevalence of at least 1.5% and all diseases included in the CCI were collected and identified using the ICD-9-CM codes. All diagnoses were extracted and coded in accordance with the method proposed by Quan et al. [10].

2.3. Study Design

The study population was divided into two different random samples in order to evaluate the accuracy of predictions and to improve the reliability of all statistical models (Figure 1):
- Training set, comprising about 50% of the subjects. All diagnoses were included in a logistic model to develop the score;
- Validation set, comprising the second half of the sample. Here, the predictive properties of the score were validated.

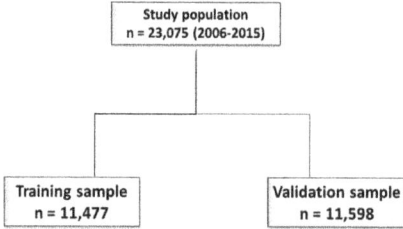

Figure 1. Flowchart of the study population.

2.4. Model Building and Statistical Analysis

Baseline information of included patients was reported as a frequency and percentage. Categorical variables were compared with a Chi-square test or Fisher's exact test, where appropriate. A multivariate logistic regression model including all diagnoses was developed to identify diagnoses associated to in-hospital mortality. All diagnoses that resulted significant were included in the final model. A weight assigned to each variable was obtained from the regression coefficient value divided by 0.3; the value obtained was rounded to the nearest integer, as proposed by Gagne et al. [11]. The PRIMOF score was calculated from the overall sum of weights. Accurate predictions discriminate between those with and those without the study outcome. Discrimination power was evaluated by estimating the C index with the 95% confidence interval. Spearman's correlation coefficient was estimated to evaluate the correlation between the CCI and PRIMOF score. Statistical significance was set to $p < 0.05$. Statistical analysis was performed by IBM SPSS Statistics v20.0 software (SPSS Inc. Chicago, IL, USA).

3. Results

During the study period, 23,075 hip-fractured patients were admitted to hospital in the Abruzzo region. Their median age (IQR) was 80.5 (69.8–89.8), and 16,749 were females (72.6%). During the hospitalization, 878 patients (3.8%) died. The training and validation samples included 11,477 and 11,598 subjects, respectively (Figure 1).

There were no significant differences between the two study groups in terms of baseline characteristics, as reported in Table 1.

Table 1. Patient characteristics.

	Training Sample (n = 11,477)	Validation Sample (n = 11,598)	*p*-Value
Age			0.817
<65	905 (7.9)	935 (8.1)	
65–85	5822 (50.7)	5899 (50.9)	
>85	4745 (41.3)	4756 (41.0)	
Female gender	8320 (72.5)	8429 (72.7)	0.755
Italian	11,311 (98.6)	11,425 (98.5)	0.835
Public Hospital	10,441 (91.0)	10,545 (90.9)	0.785
Death	433 (3.8)	445 (3.8)	0.799
Cancer	110 (1.0)	105 (0.9)	0.674
Hematologic disease	2623 (22.9)	2646 (22.8)	0.942
Ischemic heart disease	101 (0.9)	106 (0.9)	0.785
Atrial fibrillation	277 (2.4)	252 (2.2)	0.222
Dementia	305 (2.7)	328 (2.8)	0.428
COPD	269 (2.3)	230 (2.0)	0.060
Heart failure	248 (2.2)	235 (2.0)	0.475
Mild Diabetes	750 (6.5)	732 (6.3)	0.489
Uncontrolled Diabetes	179 (1.6)	183 (1.6)	0.911
Peripheral vascular disease	24 (0.2)	29 (0.3)	0.516
Cerebrovascular disease	253 (2.2)	239 (2.1)	0.450
Rheumatologic disease	31 (0.3)	32 (0.3)	0.933
Ulcer	29 (0.3)	21 (0.2)	0.242
Slight hepatic disease	98 (0.9)	83 (0.7)	0.234
Severe hepatic disease	4 (0.1)	6 (0.1)	0.988
Plegia	63 (0.5)	52 (0.4)	0.278
Kidney disease	263 (2.3)	306 (2.6)	0.151
Metastasis	30 (0.3)	30 (0.3)	0.999
HIV/AIDS	1 (0.0)	3 (0.0)	0.989

3.1. Development of PRIMOF in the Training Sample

In the training set, a logistic model was developed to assess the weights of different diagnoses. All diagnoses not significantly associated with the study outcome were excluded from the final model. Table 2 reported all regression coefficient values calculated on in-hospital mortality and relatives assigned weight.

Table 2. Assignment of weights in the development of PRIMOF score through multivariable logistic regression.

Diagnosis	Coefficient	OR (95% CI)	Weight
Age			
65–85	1.18	3.25 (1.58–6.68)	4
>85	2.09	8.06 (3.94–16.51)	7
Female gender	0.66	1.93 (1.57–2.39)	2
Cancer	1.25	3.51 (2.03–6.06)	4
Atrial fibrillation	0.52	1.68 (1.07–2.62)	2
COPD	0.58	1.79 (1.16–2.75)	6
Cerebrovascular disease	0.95	2.59 (1.67–4.01)	9
Ulcer	1.65	5.22 (1.74–15.71)	5
Kidney disease	0.95	2.58 (1.71–3.88)	3
Heart failure	1.97	7.18 (5.18–9.97)	7

PRIMOF was obtained through the sum of the different diagnosis weights. The score ranged between 0 and 45. The highest score observed among enrolled patients in the training set was 27. Due to the small number of cases, subjects with a score higher than 10 were grouped and then considered in the upper risk class. After, 12 classes of PRIMOF score were identified. The score was divided into four groups to improve the score interpretation:

— Class 1 from 0 to 3;
— Class 2 from 4 to 6;
— Class 3 from 7 to 9;
— Class 4 higher than 9.

3.2. Validation Procedure and Comparison with the Charlson Comorbidity Index

A significant increase in odds ratio was reported with the increase in PRIMOF score in the validation group, closely emulating the results showed in the training set (Table 3).

Table 3. Odds ratios for in-hospital mortality according to PRIMOF score.

Score	Training Set		Validation Set	
	OR (95% CI)	p-Value	OR (95% CI)	p-Value
0–3	ref		ref	
4–6	3.35 (1.22–9.17)	0.018	2.61 (1.21–5.62)	0.014
7–9	9.98 (3.70–26.95)	<0.001	5.71 (2.68–12.19)	<0.001
>9	40.28 (14.85–109–24)	<0.001	23.99 (11.16–51.60)	<0.001

The evaluation of accuracy was estimated via C-statistic (0.743; 95% CI 0.726–0.760; $p < 0.001$). The score reported a good calibration, with a non-significant Hosmer–Lemeshow test (Chi-squared 5.93; $p = 0.313$). PRIMOF and CCI were significantly correlated (Rho: 0.651; $p < 0.001$); however, compared to PRIMOF, CCI showed less accuracy in predicting in-hospital mortality in this sample. In particular, the C-index was 0.690 (95% CI 0.672–0.708; $p < 0.001$), as shown in Figure 2.

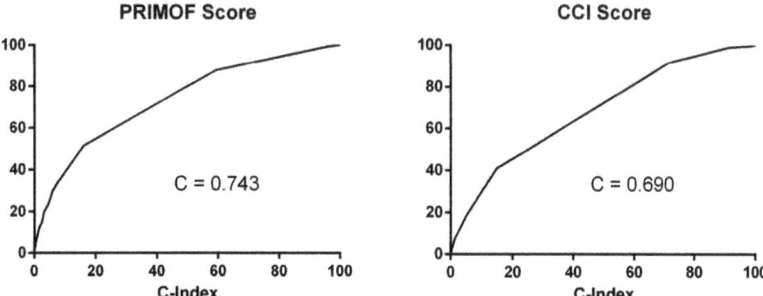

Figure 2. C-index of PRIMOF score and CCI score.

4. Discussion

4.1. Main Findings

This study demonstrates that a simple tool, based on clinical characteristics of patients, was able to stratify the risk of hip fractured population in terms of hospital mortality. In particular, the PRIMOF score performance was better than the CCI in predicting mortality among hip-fractured patients.

4.2. Comparison with Previous Studies

Many clinical risk scores were developed to predict in-hospital death of hip-fractured patients. There is a large variety of predictive tools used to identify patients at high risk through the mix of clinical and laboratory variables [12,13]. Frequently, obtaining all this information is unfeasible in many instances. Validated comorbidity indexes have also been used on admission data to predict the risk of mortality, but they were developed taking into account the general population and not hip-fractured patients. Particularly, many common scoring systems were adapted to hip fracture: ASA [14,15], CCI [16,17], and Nottingham Hip Fracture Score (NHFS) [7,17] are the most common. Additionally, the orthopedic version of POSSUM [6] was used for this aim, with Area Under the Receiver Operating Characteristic (AUROC) values ranging from 0.62 to 0.74 for mortality [12]. However, calibration showed poor results, with the observed and expected ratio ranging from 0.12 to 1.19 [12]. The NHFS and CCI use readily available pre-operative characteristics. They both have practical discriminant characteristics for mortality and were externally validated from their original cohort. The CCI was derived from well-defined variables. It is a moderately discriminant score for in-hospital morbidity and one-year mortality. However, calibration is not well reported, and this limits its capacity as audit tool. The NHFS is a hip-fracture-specific tool developed for early hospital discharge [18], 30-day mortality [7], and 1-year mortality [19]. Its discrimination ability is moderate and has good calibration. All the required items are routinely collected. Its main limitation is the use of the Abbreviated Mental Test Score (AMTS) as a cognitive impairment assessment score, which is not frequently used outside the UK [10]. In addition, NHFS did not predict in-hospital mortality.

4.3. Implications for Clinical Practice

The use of risk scores during the admission period has normally been accepted by physicians. It aims to improve clinical outcomes and service quality. The availability of a specific-disease tool able to catch the clinical complexity of admitted patients could help physicians in their daily activity. Moreover, the selection of patients at high risk of in-hospital mortality is useful for providers and healthcare services [20,21].

4.4. Strengths and Limitations

The main strength of the PRIMOF score is its reliance on a single data source, based on ICD-9-CM codes, widely used in many countries. In addition, it results in good accuracy and calibration.

The study has some limitations. Firstly, the identification of diagnosis is based on ICD-9-CM codes that do not consider the severity of reported diseases. Second, the use of HDR may be limited by the lack of certain types of information such as drug therapy. Finally, the true prevalence of some comorbidities was underestimated due to underreporting of them in the HDR.

5. Conclusions

This study showed that a simple score, based on the subject clinical history, can stratify the risk of in-hospital mortality among hip-fractured patients.

Author Contributions: Conceptualization G.D.M., F.R. and T.S.; methodology, P.S. and F.C.; software, F.C., M.D. and F.M.; validation G.D.M., P.S. and P.D.G.; formal analysis, F.C. and G.D.M.; data curation F.C., P.S. and G.D.M.; writing—original draft preparation, G.D.M., F.M. and P.S.; writing—review and editing, M.D., P.D.G., F.R. and T.S.; supervision, F.R. and T.S. All authors have read and agreed to the published version of the manuscript.

Funding: This research received no external funding.

Institutional Review Board Statement: Ethical approval was not required because the study used data that were anonymized before the analysis at the regional statistical office. Each patient was assigned to a unique identifier. The study was conducted in accord to the regulations of the Abruzzo Regional Health Authority and accordingly to the Italian Law on privacy (Art. 20-21 DL 196/2003).

Informed Consent Statement: The use of HDR did not require specific informed consent.

Data Availability Statement: Restrictions apply to the availability of these data. Data was obtained from Department of Health and Welfare of the Abruzzo region, Italy, and are available after reasonable request with the permission of the Department of Health and Welfare of the Abruzzo region.

Acknowledgments: The authors are very grateful to the Department of Health and Welfare of the Abruzzo region (Servizio Governo Dati e Flussi Informativi) for obtaining the data.

Conflicts of Interest: The authors declare no conflict of interest.

References

1. Marks, R. Hip fracture epidemiological trends, outcomes, and risk factors, 1970–2009. *Int. J. Gen. Med.* **2010**, *3*, 1–17. [CrossRef] [PubMed]
2. Aigner, R.M.F.T.; Eschbach, D.; Hack, J.; Bliemel, C.; Ruchholtz, S.; Bücking, B. Patient factors associated with increased acute care costs of hip fractures: A detailed analysis of 402 patients. *Arch. Osteoporos.* **2016**, *11*, 38. [CrossRef] [PubMed]
3. Neuhaus, V.; King, J.; Hageman, M.G.; Ring, D.C. Charlson comorbidity indices and in-hospital deaths in patients with hip fractures. *Clin. Orthop. Relat. Res.* **2013**, *471*, 1712–1719. [CrossRef] [PubMed]
4. Di Giovanni, P.; Di Martino, G.; Zecca, I.A.; Porfilio, I.; Romano, F.; Staniscia, T. Incidence of hip fracture and 30-day hospital readmissions in a region of central Italy from 2006 to 2015. *Geriatr. Gerontol. Int.* **2019**, *19*, 483–486. [CrossRef] [PubMed]
5. Charlson, M.; Szatrowski, T.P.; Peterson, J.; Gold, J. Validation of a combined comorbidity index. *J. Clin. Epidemiol.* **1994**, *47*, 1245–1251. [CrossRef]
6. Blay-Domínguez, E.; Lajara-Marco, F.; Bernáldez-Silvetti, P.F.; Veracruz-Gálvez, E.M.; Muela-Pérez, B.; Palazón-Banegas, M.Á.; Salinas-Gilabert, J.E.; Lozano-Requena, J.A. O-POSSUM score predicts morbidity and mortality in patients undergoing hip fracture surgery. *Rev. Esp. Cir. Ortop. Traumatol.* **2018**, *62*, 207–215. [CrossRef]
7. Moppett, I.K.; Parker, M.; Griffiths, R.; Bowers, T.; White, S.M.; Moran, C.G. Nottingham hip fracture score: Longitudinal and multicentre assessment. *Br. J. Anaesth.* **2012**, *109*, 546–550. [CrossRef] [PubMed]
8. Jones, H.J.; de Cossart, L. Risk scoring in surgical patients. Risk scoring in surgical patients. *Br. J. Surg.* **1999**, *86*, 149–157. [CrossRef]
9. Di Martino, G.; Di Giovanni, P.; Cedrone, F.; D'Addezio, M.; Meo, F.; Scampoli, P.; Romano, F.; Staniscia, T. The Burden of Diabetes-Related Preventable Hospitalization: 11-Year Trend and Associated Factors in a Region of Southern Italy. *Healthcare* **2021**, *9*, 997. [CrossRef] [PubMed]

10. Quan, H.; Sundararajan, V.; Halfon, P.; Fong, A.; Burnand, B.; Luthi, J.C.; Saunders, L.D.; Beck, C.A.; Feasby, T.E.; Ghali, W.A. Coding algorithms for defining comorbidities in ICD-9-CM and ICD-10 administrative data. *Med. Care* **2005**, 1130–1139. [CrossRef]
11. Gagne, J.J.; Glynn, R.J.; Avorn, J.; Levin, R.; Schneeweiss, S. A combined comorbidity score predicted mortality in elderly patients better than existing scores. *J. Clin. Epidemiol.* **2011**, *64*, 749–759. [CrossRef] [PubMed]
12. Marufu, T.C.; Mannings, A.; Moppett, I.K. Risk scoring models for predicting peri-operative morbidity and mortality in people with fragility hip fractures: Qualitative systematic review. *Injury* **2015**, *46*, 2325–2334. [CrossRef] [PubMed]
13. Di Giovanni, P.; Di Martino, G.; Zecca, I.A.L.; Porfilio, I.; Romano, F.; Staniscia, T. Predictors of Prolonged Hospitalization and In-Hospital Mortality after Hip Fracture: A Retrospective Study on Discharge Registry. *Ann Ig* **2021**. [CrossRef]
14. Burgos, E.; Gomez-Arnau, J.I.; Diez, R.; Munoz, L.; Fernandez-Guisasola, J.; del Valle, S.G. Predictive value of six risk scores for outcome after surgical repair of hip fracture in elderly patients. *Acta Anaesth. Scand.* **2008**, *52*, 125–131. [CrossRef] [PubMed]
15. Toson, B.; Harvey, L.A.; Close, J.C. The ICD-10 Charlson Comorbidity Index predicted mortality but not resource utilization following hip fracture. *J. Clin. Epidemiol.* **2015**, *68*, 44–51. [CrossRef] [PubMed]
16. Radley, D.C.; Gottlieb, D.J.; Fisher, E.S.; Tosteson, A.N.A. Comorbidity risk-adjustment strategies are comparable among persons with hip fracture. *J. Clin. Epidemiol.* **2008**, *61*, 580–587. [CrossRef]
17. Wiles, M.D.; Moran, C.G.; Sahota, O.; Moppett, I.K. Nottingham Hip Fracture Score as a predictor of one year mortality in patients undergoing surgical repair of fractured neck of femur. *Br. J. Anaesth.* **2011**, *106*, 501–504. [CrossRef]
18. Moppett, I.K.; Wiles, M.D.; Moran, C.G.; Sahota, O. The Nottingham Hip Fracture Score as a predictor of early discharge following fractured neck of femur. *Age Ageing* **2012**, *41*, 322–326. [CrossRef]
19. Maxwell, M.J.; Moran, C.G.; Moppett, I.K. Development and validation of a preoperative scoring system to predict 30 day mortality in patients undergoing hip fracture surgery. *Br. J. Anaesth.* **2008**, *101*, 511–517. [CrossRef]
20. Polder, J.J.; Barendregt, J.J.; van Oers, H. Health care costs in the last year of life—The Dutch experience. *Soc. Sci. Med.* **2006**, *63*, 1720–1731, PMID: 16781037. [CrossRef]
21. Di Giovanni, P.; Di Martino, G.; Zecca, I.A.L.; Porfilio, I.; Romano, F.; Staniscia, T. Outcomes comparison between hip fracture surgery and elective hip replacement: A propensity score-matched analysis on administrative data. *Eur. Geriatr. Med.* **2019**, *10*, 61–66. [CrossRef] [PubMed]

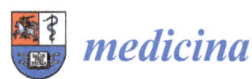

Article

Surgical Management and Outcomes Following Pathologic Hip Fracture—Results from a Propensity Matching Analysis of the Registry for Geriatric Trauma of the German Trauma Society

Christopher Bliemel [1,*], Katherine Rascher [2], Ludwig Oberkircher [3], Torsten Schlosshauer [4], Carsten Schoeneberg [5], Matthias Knobe [6], Bastian Pass [5], Steffen Ruchholtz [1], Antonio Klasan [7] and on behalf of the AltersTraumaRegister DGU [†]

1. Center for Orthopaedics and Trauma Surgery, University Hospital Giessen-Marburg, Baldingerstrasse, 35043 Marburg, Germany; ruchholt@med.uni-marburg.de
2. Akademie der Unfallchirurgie GmbH, 80538 Munich, Germany; katherine.rascher@auc-online.de
3. Department of Trauma Surgery, Orthopaedics and Arthroplasty, Hospital Friedrichshafen, 88048 Friedrichshafen, Germany; l.oberkircher@klinikum-fn.de
4. Department of Plastic Surgery, Agaplesion Evangelical Hospital Giessen, 35398 Gießen, Germany; torsten.schlosshauer@ekm-gi.de
5. Department of Orthopedic and Emergency Surgery, Alfried Krupp Hospital Essen, 45131 Essen, Germany; carsten.schoeneberg@krupp-krankenhaus.de (C.S.); bastian.pass@krupp-krankenhaus.de (B.P.)
6. Department of Orthopaedic and Trauma Surgery, Cantone Hospital Lucerne, 6004 Luzern, Switzerland; matthias.knobe@luks.ch
7. Department for Orthopaedics and Traumatology, Kepler University Hospital Linz, 4020 Linz, Austria; klasan.antonio@me.com
* Correspondence: bliemel@med.uni-marburg.de; Tel.: +49-6421-58-66216
† Working Committee on Geriatric Trauma Registry (AK ATR) of the German Trauma Society (DGU).

Abstract: *Background and Objectives:* The outcomes of patients with pathologic hip fractures remain unclear. Data from a large international geriatric trauma registry were analyzed to examine the outcomes of patients with pathologic hip fractures compared with patients with typical osteoporotic hip fractures. *Materials and Methods:* Data from the Registry for Geriatric Trauma of the German Trauma Society (Deutsche Gesellschaft für Unfallchirurgie (DGU)) (ATR-DGU) were analyzed. All patients treated surgically for osteoporotic or pathologic hip fractures were included in this analysis. Across both fracture types, a 2:1 optimal propensity score matching and multivariate logistic regression analysis were conducted. In-house mortality rate and mortality at the 120-day follow-up, as well as mobility after 7 and 120 days, reoperation rate, discharge management from the hospital and readmission rate to the hospital until the 120-day follow-up were analyzed as outcome parameters for the underlying fracture type—pathologic or osteoporotic. *Results:* A total of 29,541 cases met the inclusion criteria. Of the patients included, 29,330 suffered from osteoporotic fractures, and 211 suffered from pathologic fractures. Multivariate logistic regression analysis revealed no differences between the two fracture types in terms of mortality during the acute hospital stay, reoperation during the initial acute hospital stay, walking ability after seven days and the likelihood of being discharged back home. Walking ability and hospital readmission remained insignificant at the 120-day follow-up as well. However, the odds of passing away within the first 120 days were significantly higher for patients suffering from pathologic hip fractures (OR: 3.07; $p = 0.003$). *Conclusions:* Surgical treatment of pathologic hip fractures was marked by a more frequent use of arthroplasty in per- and subtrochanteric fractures. Furthermore, the mortality rate among patients suffering from pathologic hip fractures was elevated in the midterm. The complication rate, as indicated by the rate of readmission to the hospital and the necessity for reoperation, remained unaffected.

Keywords: pathologic femoral fracture; outcome; mortality; mobility; AltersTraumaRegister DGU®

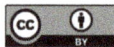

1. Introduction

In comparison to traumatic bone fractures, pathologic fractures due to diseased bone are less common events. A pathologic fracture is one that occurs without adequate trauma and is in most cases caused by a malignant bony lesion. Apart from primary malignant osseous tumors, osseous metastasizing carcinomas of the lung, breast, kidney, thyroid gland and prostate are responsible for the vast majority of bony lesions [1]. Apart from prostate metastases, which are usually osteoblastic, bony lesions mainly appear as lytic or mixed.

Due to a very well-developed vascular system in the intertrochanteric region, bony metastases are particularly common in the area of the proximal femur [2,3]. This circumstance favors pathologic fractures of the hip, as the mechanical loading stress during walking, which is transferred from the pelvic ring on to the femoral shaft, is extremely high [4–8].

As the vast majority of geriatric hip fractures are known to be related to osteoporosis rather than cancer, it is scarcely surprising that most of the literature focuses on this primary cause [9–11]. Such findings on geriatric hip fractures have already been included in national guidelines for several years and are further implemented as quality indicators in the treatment of geriatric hip fracture patients [12,13].

Despite the overlap between both patient groups with regard to fracture site and therapeutic goals, such as pain relief, mobilization or maintenance of patients' independence, it remains unclear whether the findings derived from osteoporotic hip fractures can be transferred one-to-one to patients with pathologic hip fractures.

Currently, the literature on this topic remains limited and contradictory. Some studies report similarities between both groups of patients, especially in terms of the occurrence of perioperative complications, such as pneumonia, wound healing disorders and sepsis [2] or in the rate of total hip arthroplasties (THAs) performed [14]. On the other hand, discordant findings were found in other studies, such as the sex rate of patients affected [15], the comorbidity profile of patients [14] or the outcome related to delay in time to surgery [16].

To provide more clarity regarding outcomes of patients with pathologic and non-pathologic fractures, we made use of the data contained in the Registry for Geriatric Trauma (AltersTraumaRegister DGU® (ATR-DGU)) of the German Trauma Society (Deutsche Gesellschaft für Unfallchirurgie (DGU)).

It was hypothesized that, compared to osteoporosis-related hip fractures, the presence of metastasis-related hip fractures would lead to increased rates of perioperative complications and mortality among those patients with pathologic fractures.

2. Materials and Methods

This study is a retrospective cohort registry study comparing patients with malignant, pathologic fractures vs. patients with non-pathologic (osteoporotic) fractures. All patient data were obtained from the ATR-DGU.

2.1. ATR-DGU

The source of the data in the present analysis is the ATR-DGU (http://www.alterstraumaregister-dgu.de (accessed on 29 November 2021). The ATR-DGU was established in 2016 by the German Trauma Society (DGU). It is a large, prospective, multicenter, standardized registry that provides information on geriatric trauma patients with hip, periprosthetic and peri-implant femoral fractures. The reliability of ATR-DGU has already been shown elsewhere [17]. All DGU-certified AltersTraumaZentren (Specialty Orthogeriatric Departments) are required to enter patient data into the ATR-DGU. Data entry was only possible with consent of the patient. Therefore, all patients who did not sign a consent form were excluded. Participating centers transmit pseudonymized patient data via a web-based application into a central database. Currently, approximately 120 hospitals from Germany, Switzerland and Austria contribute to the ATR-DGU. The scientific management of the ATR-DGU is carried out by the Working Committee on Geriatric Trauma Registry (AK

ATR) of the DGU. Approval for scientific data analysis from the ATR-DGU is granted via a peer-review process in accordance with the publication guidelines laid out by the AK ATR. The present study is in accordance with the publication guidelines of the ATR-DGU and registered as ATR-DGU project ID 2021-007. The inclusion criteria of the ATR-DGU are patients with proximal femur fractures, including periprosthetic and peri-implant fractures requiring surgery, who are aged 70 years or older. The ATR-DGU collects data in five distinct phases: pre-injury, intake, surgery, first week post-surgery and an optional 120-day follow-up [18].

2.2. Inclusion and Exclusion Criteria

This study analyzed 34,895 patients documented in the registry from 2016 to 2020. Patients with periprosthetic and peri-implant fractures were excluded, as well as atypical femoral fractures and fractures of unknown entity. This resulted in an initial analysis group of 29,541 patients from 119 hospitals. Two patient groups were compared—those with malignant, pathologic fractures vs. patients with non-pathologic (osteoporotic) fractures. Outcome parameters were mortality during the acute hospital stay and until the 120-day follow-up, reoperation rate during the initial hospital stay, walking ability 7 and 120 days after surgery, living situation after release from the hospital and readmission to the hospital during the follow-up phase.

2.3. Statistical Analysis

To control for differences between the demographics of the two groups, a 2:1 optimal propensity score matching was conducted. Matching was performed using the MatchIt package [19] in R v. 4.0.2 (Foundation for Statistical Computing, Vienna, Austria), which uses functions from the optmatch package [20]. The covariates used in the matching were age, sex, American Society of Anesthesiologists (ASA) score, type of fracture and walking ability before fracture. After matching, the absolute standardized mean differences of all covariates were less than 0.08, indicating that good balance was achieved.

For descriptive analyses, categorical data are presented as counts and percentages, and continuous variables are presented as the means with standard deviation (sd). Comparisons between patient groups were made using the χ^2-test for categorical variables and the Mann–Whitney test for continuous variables. Furthermore, logistic and linear regressions were performed on the matched dataset to test for differences in the above-listed outcome parameters. All differences were considered statistically significant when $p < 0.05$.

2.4. Aim of the Study and Outcome Parameters

The aim of the study was to analyze the differences in complication and mortality rates during the acute hospital stay and at the 120-day follow-up, depending on the fracture type—pathologic or non-pathologic (osteoporotic). Univariable outcomes were examined separately for patients who suffered from non-pathologic and pathologic hip fractures (Figure 1). Other outcomes studied were the mobility of patients, their reoperation rate and discharge management, as well as the rate of readmission to the hospital within the first 120 days following the initial surgical treatment.

The present analysis covered the following data: sex, age, ASA score, Identification of Seniors At Risk (ISAR) score [21], residential status (before the fracture and at 120-day follow-up), fracture type, anticoagulation on admission, time to surgery, type of surgical treatment, surgical complication (120-day follow-up), walking ability (on day 7 after surgery and at 120-day follow-up), discharge after hospital and mortality (at the initial stay and at 120-day follow-up).

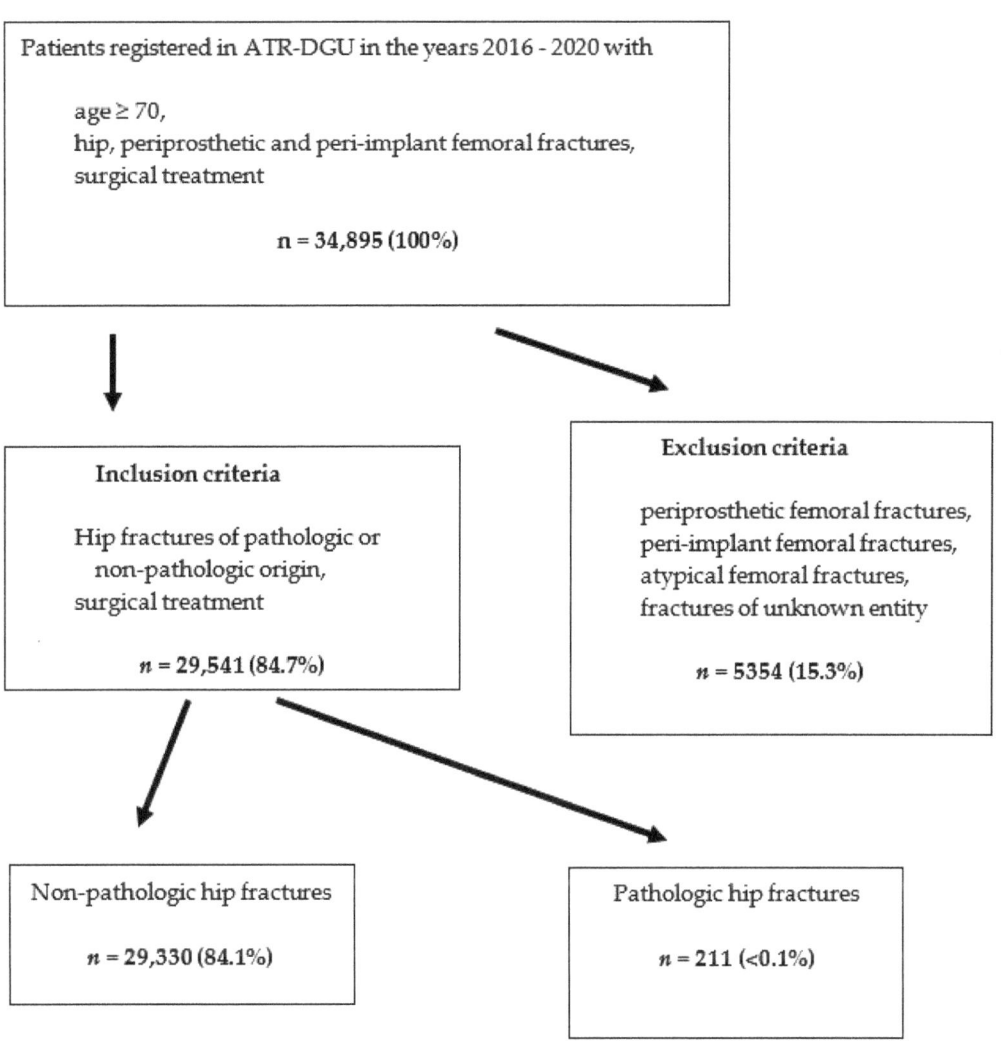

Figure 1. Flow sheet of the included population.

3. Results

3.1. Acute Care Data

A total of 29,541 hip fractures from geriatric trauma patients met the inclusion criteria. Of these fractures, 29,330 fractures were of non-pathologic origin, and 211 fractures were of pathologic origin.

Univariable data analysis in terms of the fracture origin (non-pathologic or pathologic) is shown in Table 1. This analysis revealed that patients with pathologic femoral fractures had a more balanced sex distribution ($p < 0.001$) and were younger in age ($p < 0.001$) than those with non-pathologic femoral fractures. Further differences were seen in the ASA score and time to surgery, with patients suffering from pathologic fractures having increased ASA scores ($p < 0.001$) and a delay in surgical stabilization ($p = 0.002$). Representing approximately a quarter of cases, subtrochanteric fractures were much more common in patients with pathologic fractures ($p < 0.001$). Patients with pathologic femoral fractures were also more likely to have an independent residential status before the fracture ($p < 0.001$) and were discharged home more often ($p = 0.002$).

Table 1. Univariable analysis of unmatched data on geriatric trauma patients with hip fractures depending on the kind of fracture entity.

Parameter		Non-Pathologic Fracture	Pathologic Fracture	p-Value
Number of patients		29,330	211	
Gender	Male	8397 (28.0%)	93 (44.1%)	<0.001 *
	Female	21,081 (72.0%)	118 (55.9%)	
Patient age (year) Mean (sd)		84.4 (6.5)	81.0 (6.7)	<0.001 **
ASA score	1	347 (1.2%)	0 (0.0%)	<0.001 *
	2	6489 (22.5%)	26 (12.5%)	
	3	19,780 (68.6%)	147 (70.7%)	
	4 and 5	2201 (7.6%)	35 (16.8%)	
ISAR score	0	2482 (11.3%)	13 (8.2%)	0.161 *
	1	2744 (12.5%)	19 (12.0%)	
	2	4775 (21.8%)	25 (15.8%)	
	3	5244 (23.9%)	40 (25.3%)	
	4	4336 (19.8%)	44 (27.8%)	
	5	1846 (8.4%)	13 (8.2%)	
	6	524 (2.4%)	4 (2.5%)	
Anticoagulatory drugs	Yes	15,387 (54.2%)	93 (45.4%)	0.014 *
	No	12,984 (45.8%)	112 (54.6%)	
Pre-fracture residential status	At home	21,802 (75.6%)	170 (82.1%)	<0.001 *
	Nursing home	6529 (22.7%)	26 (12.6%)	
	Hospital	361 (1.3%)	9 (4.3%)	
	Other	133 (0.5%)	2 (1.0%)	
Fracture type	Hip fracture	13,767 (47.0%)	86 (41.1%)	<0.001 *
	Trochanteric fracture	14,359 (49.0%)	70 (33.5%)	
	Subtrochanteric fracture	1166 (4.0%)	53 (25.4%)	
Time to surgery (h)	<12 h	10,849 (37.3%)	67 (32.2%)	0.002 *
	12–24 h	10,466 (35.9%)	65 (31.2%)	
	24–36 h	3755 (12.9%)	29 (13.9%)	
	24–48 h	1888 (6.5%)	17 (8.2%)	
	>48	2157 (7.4%)	30 (14.4%)	
Type of surgical treatment +	Total hip arthroplasty	2389	24	
	Hemiarthroplasty	10,136	65	
	Trochanteric nail	14,742	102	
	Dynamic hip screw	929	10	
	Cannulates screw	381	2	
	Other	913	11	
Pre-fracture walking ability	Independent without walking aids	9610 (35.1%)	57 (29.1%)	0.158 *
	Ability to walk outside with a walking stick or crutch	3296 (12.1%)	34 (17.3%)	
	Ability to walk outside with two crutches or a walker	8882 (32.5%)	64 (32.7%)	
	Certain walking ability in the apartment, but outside only with an assistant	4694 (17.2%)	35 (17.9%)	
	No functional walking ability	869 (3.2%)	6 (3.1%)	
Death during stay in the acute hospital	Yes	1622 (5.5%)	22 (10.4%)	0.065 *
	No	27,649 (94.5%)	189 (89.6%)	

Table 1. Cont.

Parameter		Non-Pathologic Fracture	Pathologic Fracture	p-Value
Ability to walk at the seventh postoperative day	Unknown	842 (2.9%)	4 (1.9%)	0.602 *
	Without aid	182 (0.6%)	3 (1.4%)	
	With walking stick or crutch	3106 (10.7%)	22 (10.6%)	
	With a rollator	8561 (29.5%)	67 (32.2%)	
	With a walking frame (no wheels)	4043 (13.9%)	29 (13.9%)	
	With a walker	6282 (21.7%)	38 (18.3%)	
	Not possible	5994 (20.7%)	45 (21.6%)	
Reoperation during initial acute hospital stay	Yes	964 (3.3%)	9 (4.3%)	0.550 *
	No	28,340 (96.7%)	202 (95.7%)	
Discharge from hospital	At home	6774 (24.8%)	57 (31.0%)	0.002 *
	Nursing home	7367 (27.0%)	38 (20.7%)	
	Inpatient stay	13,151 (48.2%)	89 (48.3%)	

* Chi-Square Test; ** Mann–Whitney; + multiple choices possible.

Due to such differences in the demographics of the baseline parameters in both patient groups, an optimal propensity score matching analysis was performed, as illustrated in Table 2. Based on a 2:1 matching of 382 patients with non-pathologic fractures and 191 patients with pathologic fractures, there was a significant delay in time to surgery for patients with pathologic fractures ($p = 0.005$). Additionally, there were significant differences in the type of surgical treatment for per- and subtrochanteric fractures, with pathologic fractures being more often treated by arthroplasty compared to non-pathologic femoral hip fractures ($p = 0.002$).

Table 2. Univariable analysis of a 2:1 optimal propensity score matching analysis of data on geriatric trauma patients with hip fractures depending on the kind of fracture entity.

Parameter		Non-Pathologic Fracture	Pathologic Fracture	p-Value
Number of patients		382	191	
Gender	Male	180 (47.1%)	83 (43.5%)	0.459 *
	Female	202 (52.9%)	108 (56.5%)	
Patient age (year) Mean (sd)		81.1 (6.6)	81.1 (6.7)	0.968 **
ASA score	2	41 (10.7%)	24 (12.6%)	0.703 *
	3	273 (71.5%)	137 (71.7%)	
	4	68 (17.8%)	30 (15.7%)	
ISAR score	0	24 (8.7%)	13 (9.0%)	0.420 *
	1	27 (9.8%)	19 (13.2%)	
	2	67 (24.3%)	22 (15.3%)	
	3	71 (25.7%)	36 (25.0%)	
	4	60 (21.7%)	39 (27.1%)	
	5	23 (8.3%)	12 (8.3%)	
	6	4 (1.4%)	3 (2.1%)	
Anticoagulatory drugs	Yes	225 (60.3%)	85 (45.5%)	0.001 *
	No	148 (39.7%)	102 (54.5%)	
Pre-fracture residential status	At home	298 (79.3%)	153 (81.0%)	0.105 *
	Nursing home	68 (18.1%)	26 (13.8%)	
	Hospital	5 (1.3%)	8 (4.2%)	
	Other	5 (1.3%)	2 (1.1%)	

Table 2. Cont.

Parameter		Non-Pathologic Fracture	Pathologic Fracture	p-Value
Fracture type	Hip fracture	163 (42.7%)	79 (41.4%)	0.814 *
	Trochanteric fracture	138 (36.1%)	67 (35.1%)	
	Subtrochanteric fracture	81 (21.2%)	45 (23.5%)	
Time to surgery (h)	<12 h	151 (39.7%)	62 (33.0%)	0.005 *
	12–24 h	152 (40.0%)	60 (31.9%)	
	24–36 h	31 (8.2%)	27 (14.4%)	
	36–48 h	21 (5.5%)	16 (8.5%)	
	≥48	25 (6.6%)	23 (12.2%)	
Type of surgical treatment +	Total hip arthroplasty	45	20	
	Hemiarthroplasty	109	60	
	Trochanteric nail	212	94	
	Dynamic hip screw	9	9	
	Cannulates screw	4	1	
	Other	10	9	
Type of surgical treatment for per- and subtrochanteric fractures	Total hip arthroplasty or hemiarthroplasty	3 (1.3%)	10 (8.8%)	0.002 *
	Osteosynthesis	221 (98.7%)	104 (91.2%)	
Pre-fracture walking ability	Independent without walking aids	106 (27.7%)	53 (27.7%)	0.892 *
	Ability to walk outside with a walking stick or crutch	62 (16.2%)	34 (17.8%)	
	Ability to walk outside with two crutches or a walker	127 (33.2%)	63 (33.0%)	
	Certain walking ability in the apartment, but outside only with an assistant	79 (20.7%)	35 (18.3%)	
	No functional walking ability	8 (2.1%)	6 (3.1%)	
Death during stay in the acute hospital	Yes	25 (6.6%)	19 (9.9%)	0.756 *
	No	356 (93.4%)	172 (90.1%)	
Ability to walk at the seventh postoperative day	Unknown	6 (1.6%)	4 (2.1%)	0.198 *
	Without aid	4 (1.1%)	2 (1.1%)	
	With walking stick or crutch	36 (9.5%)	22 (11.6%)	
	With a rollator	120 (31.7%)	61 (32.3%)	
	With a walking frame (no wheels)	37 (9.8%)	29 (15.3%)	
	With a walker	103 (27.2%)	34 (18.0%)	
	Not possible	72 (19.0%)	37 (19.6%)	
Reoperation during initial acute hospital stay	Yes	10 (2.6%)	8 (4.2%)	0.446 *
	No	372 (97.4%)	183 (95.8%)	
Discharge from hospital	At home	92 (25.9%)	54 (32.3%)	0.202 *
	Nursing home	86 (24.2%)	36 (21.6%)	
	Inpatient stay	177 (49.9%)	77 (46.1%)	

* Chi-Square Test; ** Mann–Whitney; + multiple choices possible.

After controlling for age, sex, ASA score, type of fracture and walking ability before fracture, no differences were found between patients with pathologic and non-pathologic hip fractures regarding death during the acute hospital stay ($p = 0.155$), the reoperation rate during the acute hospital stay ($p = 0.314$), the walking ability after seven days ($p = 0.856$) or being discharged back home rather than to an inpatient facility ($p = 0.295$) (Table 3).

3.2. 120-Day Follow-Up Data

For 12,887 patients with non-pathologic hip fractures and 86 patients with pathologic hip fractures, data are available at the time of the 120-day follow-up (Table 4).

Patients suffering from pathologic fractures had a significantly higher mortality rate within the first 120 days following surgery compared to non-pathologic hip fracture patients (31% vs. 11%; $p = 0.001$). Other parameters, such as walking ability ($p = 0.588$), place of residence ($p = 0.965$), preoperative vs. postoperative change in residential status ($p = 0.988$) and the rate of readmission or reoperation during the follow-up period ($p = 0.648$ and $p = 0.374$), were comparable between both fracture types (Table 4).

Based on a 2:1 matching, 138 non-pathologic hip fracture patients were compared to 84 patients with pathologic hip fractures. Trends in the matched data were the same as those in the unmatched data. Mortality was significantly higher in the pathologic fracture group than in the non-pathologic fracture group ($p < 0.001$). In contrast, place of residence did not differ significantly across the two fracture groups ($p = 0.965$). Similarly, there were no significant differences in patients' ability to walk ($p = 0.627$), the preoperative vs. postoperative change in residence ($p = 0.903$) or the rate of readmission or reoperation during the follow-up period ($p = 0.920$ and $p = 0.725$; Table 5).

Multivariate analysis of parameters collected at follow-up showed that the odds ratio for dying within 120 days postoperatively was significantly higher in patients with pathologic fractures (OR: 3.07; $p = 0.003$; Table 3). However, the 120-day readmission rate and patients' walking ability did not differ between patients with non-pathologic and pathologic fractures ($p = 0.683$ and $p = 0.396$) (Table 3).

Table 3. Multivariable logistic regression analysis—pathologic vs. non-pathologic femur fracture. Analysis is adjusted for sex, patient age, ASA score, fracture type and pre-fracture walking ability. The model "discharge from hospital" is adjusted to the pre-fracture living situation.

Influence of the Fracture Entity on ...	N	OR	95%-CI and OR	p-Value
Acute phase				
Death during stay in the acute hospital * Yes vs. no	573	1.57	[0.83; 2.92]	0.155
Reoperation during initial acute hospital stay * Yes vs. no	573	1.63	[0.61; 4.19]	0.314
Walking ability after seven days * able to walk vs. not able/only at home	557	0.96	[0.62; 1.51]	0.856
Discharge from hospital back home * Yes vs. no	519	1.25	[0.82; 1.91]	0.295
120-day follow-up				
Mortality during follow-up * Yes vs. no	222	3.07	[1.46; 6.47]	0.003
Readmission to hospital during follow-up * Yes vs. no	213	1.28	[0.39; 4.18]	0.683
Walking ability after 120 days * able to walk vs. not able/only at home	175	0.64	[0.23; 1.86]	0.396

* Logistic regression.

Table 4. Univariable analysis of 120-day follow-up data on geriatric trauma patients with hip fractures depending on the kind of fracture entity.

Parameter		Non-Pathologic Fracture	Pathologic Fracture	p-Value
Number of patients		12,887	86	
Ability to walk	Without aid	1044 (10.9%)	4 (7.0%)	0.588 *
	With walking stick or crutch	1153 (12.1%)	9 (15.8%)	
	With two crutches or a rollator	4069 (42.6%)	28 (49.1%)	
	Certain ability to walk indoors	2020 (21.1%)	9 (15.8%)	
	Not possible	1270 (13.3%)	7 (12.3%)	
Residential status	At home\assisted living facility	6008 (67.1%)	36 (76.6%)	<0.361 *
	Nursing home	2768 (30.9%)	10 (21.3%)	
	Hospital\Inpatient Facility	178 (2.0%)	1 (2.1%)	
120-day mortality	Dead	1122 (11%)	21 (30.9%)	<0.001 *
Changes in living situation at 120-day follow-up	Pre-fracture living at home and still living at home	5666 (82.4%)	34 (82.9%)	0.988 *
	Pre-fracture living at home changed to nursing home	1056 (15.4%)	6 (14.6%)	
	Pre-fracture living at home changed to other inpatient facility	152 (2.2%)	1 (2.4)	
Readmission to hospital during follow-up	Yes	569 (4.6%)	5 (6.3%)	0.648 *
	No	11,774 (95.4%)	74 (93.7%)	
Reoperation during follow-up	Yes	469 (4.0%)	5 (6.7%)	0.374 *
	No	11,315 (96.0%)	70 (93.3%)	
Type of reoperation +	Conversion into total hip arthroplasty	81	0	
	Conversion into hemiarthroplasty	51	0	
	Girdlestone situation	9	0	
	Periprosthetic fracture/peri-implant fracture	42	0	
	Implant removal	84	0	
	Reposition	45	?	
	Revision of osteosynthesis	57	1	
	Irrigation or debridement	130	2	
	Other	115	1	

* Chi-Square Test; + multiple choices possible.

Table 5. Univariable analysis of a 2:1 optimal propensity score matching analysis of 120-day follow-up data on geriatric trauma patients with hip fractures depending on the kind of fracture entity.

Parameter		Non-Pathologic Fracture	Pathologic Fracture	p-Value
Number of patients		138	84	
Ability to walk	Without aid	13 (10.9%)	4 (7.1%)	0.627 *
	With walking stick or crutch	14 (11.8%)	9 (16.1%)	
	With two crutches or a rollator	55 (46.2%)	27 (48.2%)	
	Certain ability to walk indoors	27 (22.7%)	9 (16.1%)	
	Not possible	10 (8.4%)	7 (12.5%)	

Table 5. Cont.

Parameter		Non-Pathologic Fracture	Pathologic Fracture	p-Value
Residential status	At home\assisted living	83 (74.8%)	35 (76.1%)	0.965 *
	Nursing home	26 (23.4%)	10 (21.7%)	
	Inpatient Facility	2 (1.8%)	1 (2.2%)	
120-day mortality	Dead	14 (11.2%)	21 (31.3%)	0.001 *
Changes in living situation at 120-day follow-up	Pre-fracture living at home and still living at home	77 (85.6%)	33 (82.5%)	0.903 *
	Pre-fracture living at home changed to nursing home	11 (12.2%)	6 (15.0%)	
	Pre-fracture living at home changed to other inpatient facility	2 (2.2%)	1 (2.5%)	
Readmission to hospital during follow-up	Yes	7 (5.1%)	5 (6.5%)	0.920 *
	No	129 (94.9%)	72 (93.5%)	
Reoperation during follow-up	Yes	6 (4.6%)	5 (6.8%)	0.725 *
	No	124 (95.4%)	68 (93.2%)	
Type of reoperation +	Conversion into total hip arthroplasty	2	0	
	Conversion into hemiarthroplasty	1	0	
	Implant removal	2	0	
	Reposition	0	2	
	Revision of osteosynthesis	1	1	
	Irrigation or debridement	0	2	
	Other	1	1	

* Chi-Square Test; + multiple choices possible.

4. Discussion

This study analyzed the surgical management and complication and mortality rate of patients with pathologic hip fractures in contrast to patients with osteoporotic hip fractures. Based on a 2:1 propensity matching, the principal findings revealed that surgical treatment differed significantly between both groups of patients. Patients suffering from pathologic per- and subtrochanteric fractures were more often treated by arthroplasty. In addition, the time to surgery was delayed in patients with pathologic femoral fractures. In terms of survival, an increased mortality rate within the first 120 days of follow-up was seen for pathologic hip fractures according to a multivariate regression analysis. Nevertheless, walking ability and complication rate, as indicated by the rates of reoperation and readmission back to hospital during the 120-day follow-up period, remained unaffected by the fracture type.

Concerning the surgical treatment strategy for pathologic hip fractures, several authors point out the value of an endoprosthetic replacement [22–24]. Having conducted a retrospective analysis of 158 patients with pertrochanteric metastatic lesions, Harvey et al. showed that endoprostheses demonstrate a lower mechanical failure rate and a higher rate of implant survivorship without mechanical failure than intramedullary nails [22]. Similar results were published by Steensma et al., who reported the clinical course of 298 patients treated surgically for impending or displaced fractures above the femoral isthmus, excluding the femoral neck. Additionally, in their patients collective, endoprosthetic reconstruction was associated with fewer treatment failures and greater implant durability [23]. Given the results from the above-named literature, it is scarcely surprising that the present registry analysis found a significantly increased rate of arthroplasties performed for per- and subtrochanteric femoral fractures. Nonetheless, with endoprosthetic replacement performed in approximately 9% of cases, the rate of endoprosthetic replacement in ATR-DGU is far below that of Steensma et al., who reported rates between 27 and 41%, depending on the individual fracture site [23].

In contrast to osteoporotic hip fractures, the time to surgery for pathologic hip fractures was significantly delayed in the present registry analysis. While surgical treatment was performed in approximately 80% of patients with osteoporotic hip fractures within the first 24 h, this was the case in only approximately 65% of patients with a pathologic fracture. While delay in time to surgery is known to be directly correlated with mortality in patients with osteoporotic hip fractures, the delay in patients suffering from pathologic femoral fractures was not associated with an increased mortality rate during the acute hospital stay in the present analysis [25]. Therefore, it must be presumed that pathologic hip fractures in geriatric patients are—other than fractures in osteoporosis-related hips—not a typical frailty marker, as is already known from other hip fracture types, e.g., periprosthetic femoral fractures [26].

Even though the mortality rate at the acute hospital stay remained unaffected by fracture type, the results of the present analysis revealed an almost three-fold increased mortality rate for patients suffering from pathologic fractures in the midterm (11.2% vs. 31.3%). Therefore, the results of this present analysis are in line with those of Amen et al., who reported on patients suffering from pathologic hip fractures with a follow-up of 30 days [2]. Based on this elevated mortality rate, Amen et al. concluded that there should be better preoperative patient counseling and shared decision making regarding the decision to undergo surgery at all. According to the results of the present study, it must be presumed that the differences in mortality rate registered among the present follow-up data are mainly driven by the natural course of the disease itself, as the follow-up period is extended up to day 120. Different to Amen et al., we believe that for patients with pathologic hip fractures, surgical fracture fixation is essential to provide adequate pain relief, mobilization and dignity until the end of life. Therefore, we advocate a consequent surgical treatment also in those patients.

In terms of mobilization and complication rates, as indicated by the rates of reoperation and readmission back to the hospital during the 120-day follow-up period, no differences were found between the fracture groups in the present ATR-DGU analysis. Therefore, our results are contradictory to those of Amen et al., who found increased rates of readmission in a 30-day follow-up period for patients with pathologic fractures vs. patients with osteoporotic hip fractures (8.4% vs. 11.9%). Differences in the rate of readmission might be related to the smaller sample size in the present study. Nevertheless, also in our analysis, an at least numerically increased rate of readmission was noticed (4.6% vs. 6.3%). Interestingly, the rates of readmission in the present analysis were much lower than those reported by Amen et al. and Varady et al., although their analyses covered a much shorter follow-up period [2,27]. In this context, it is worth noting that all patients included in this analysis were treated in certified orthogeriatric trauma centers. These centers provide access to orthogeriatric co-management under the best possible conditions that might also cushion the negative effects presumed for patients suffering from cancer-associated as well as osteoporosis-associated hip fractures [28].

Limitations

Because the present analysis is based on registry data, some limitations must be recognized. While well-designed randomized trials can prove causality, registry analyses, such as the present one, can only describe associations. Our findings must therefore be interpreted with caution. The fact that there is a certain heterogeneity in the patient population included further tempers these findings, as there are different kinds of cancer responsible for the patients subsumed in the group with pathological femoral fractures. Furthermore, due to limitations of the standard documentation sheet thus far, it remains unknown whether the fractures are due to metastases or primary malignant tumors. A possible revision of the standard documentation sheet could allow a more precise statement on this issue in the future.

Despite these above-mentioned limitations, the overall high number of participants included strengthens the results of this registry analysis. Furthermore, with the inclusion of patients from multiple geriatric trauma centers all over Germany, Switzerland and Austria, the present study provides a comprehensive overview of the current treatment strategies and outcomes related to pathologic hip fractures in central Europe.

5. Conclusions

The results of the present registry analysis further support current research, as they reveal that outcomes between pathologic and osteoporotic hip fractures are different in terms of surgical treatment strategies, time to surgery and mortality rate in the midterm. The complication rate, as indicated by the rate of readmission to the hospital and the necessity for reoperation, as well as the patients' walking ability, remained unaffected in the present analysis.

Author Contributions: C.B. contributed to the literature search, study design, data interpretation and writing of the manuscript, and approved the submitted version of the manuscript. K.R. contributed to the study design, data analysis and data interpretation, and approved the submitted version of the manuscript. L.O. contributed to the literature search, critical revision and data interpretation, and approved the submitted version of the manuscript. T.S. contributed to the literature search, critical revision and data interpretation, and approved the submitted version of the manuscript. C.S. contributed to the literature search, critical revision and data interpretation, and approved the submitted version of the manuscript. M.K. contributed to the critical revision, data interpretation and approved the submitted version of the manuscript. B.P. contributed to the data interpretation and approved the submitted version of the manuscript. S.R. contributed to the literature search, study design and data interpretation, and approved the submitted version of the manuscript. A.K. contributed to the literature search, critical revision and data interpretation, and approved the submitted version of the manuscript. All authors have read and agreed to the published version of the manuscript.

Funding: This research received no external funding. No additional financial support for the execution of the study was received.

Institutional Review Board Statement: The study was conducted according to the guidelines of the Declaration of Helsinki and approved by the Ethics Committee of Philipps-University Marburg (Ethical Approval Code: AZ 46/16).

Informed consent statement: Informed consent was obtained from all subjects involved in the study.

Data Availability Statement: Not applicable.

Conflicts of Interest: The corresponding author declares, on behalf of all the authors, that there are no conflicts of interest.

References

1. Bliemel, C.; Buecking, B.; Oberkircher, L.; Knobe, M.; Ruchholtz, S.; Eschbach, D. The impact of pre-existing conditions on functional outcome and mortality in geriatric hip fracture patients. *Int. Orthop.* **2017**, *41*, 1995–2000. [CrossRef]
2. Amen, T.B.; Varady, N.H.; Hayden, B.L.; Chen, A.F. Pathologic Versus Native Hip Fractures: Comparing 30-day Mortality and Short-term Complication Profiles. *J. Arthroplast.* **2020**, *35*, 1194–1199. [CrossRef] [PubMed]
3. Guzik, G. Oncological and functional results after surgical treatment of bone metastases at the proximal femur. *BMC Surg.* **2018**, *18*, 5. [CrossRef] [PubMed]
4. Bliemel, C.; Anrich, D.; Knauf, T.; Oberkircher, L.; Eschbach, D.; Klasan, A.; Debus, F.; Ruchholtz, S.; Bäumlein, M. More than a reposition tool: Additional wire cerclage leads to increased load to failure in plate osteosynthesis for supracondylar femoral shaft fractures. *Arch. Orthop. Trauma. Surg.* **2020**, *141*, 1197–1205. [CrossRef] [PubMed]
5. Bergmann, G.; Deuretzbacher, G.; Heller, M.; Graichen, F.; Rohlmann, A.; Strauss, J.; Duda, G. Hip contact forces and gait patterns from routine activities. *J. Biomech.* **2001**, *34*, 859–871. [CrossRef]
6. Bliemel, C.; Buecking, B.; Mueller, T.; Wack, C.; Koutras, C.; Beck, T.; Ruchholtz, S.; Zettl, R. Distal femoral fractures in the elderly: Biomechanical analysis of a polyaxial angle-stable locking plate versus a retrograde intramedullary nail in a human cadaveric bone model. *Arch. Orthop. Trauma. Surg.* **2014**, *135*, 49–58. [CrossRef]

7. Bliemel, C.; Oberkircher, L.; Bockmann, B.; Petzold, E.; Aigner, R.; Heyse, T.J.; Ruchholtz, S.; Buecking, B. Impact of cement-augmented condylar screws in locking plate osteosynthesis for distal femoral fractures—A biomechanical analysis. *Injury* **2016**, *47*, 2688–2693. [CrossRef]
8. Bäumlein, M.; Klasan, A.; Klötzer, C.; Bockmann, B.; Eschbach, D.; Knobe, M.; Bücking, B.; Ruchholtz, S.; Bliemel, C. Cement augmentation of an angular stable plate osteosynthesis for supracondylar femoral fractures-biomechanical investigation of a new fixation device. *BMC Musculoskelet. Disord.* **2020**, *21*, 1–9. [CrossRef]
9. Bliemel, C.; Bieneck, F.; Riem, S.; Hartwig, E.; Liener, U.C.; Ruchholtz, S.; Buecking, B. Subsequent treatment following proximal femoral fracture—Who, when, where? Assessment of the current situation in Germany. *Z. Orthop. Unfall.* **2012**, *150*, 210–217. [CrossRef]
10. Bliemel, C.; Oberkircher, L.; Eschbach, D.A.; Struewer, J.; Ruchholtz, S.; Buecking, B. Surgical treatment of proximal femoral fractures—A training intervention? *Z. Orthop. Unfall.* **2013**, *151*, 180–188.
11. Bliemel, C.; Sielski, R.; Doering, B.; Dodel, R.; Balzer-Geldsetzer, M.; Ruchholtz, S.; Buecking, B. Pre-fracture quality of life predicts 1-year survival in elderly patients with hip fracture—Development of a new scoring system. *Osteoporos. Int.* **2016**, *27*, 1979–1987. [CrossRef] [PubMed]
12. Liener, U.; Becker, C.; Rapp, K. *Weissbuch Alterstraumatologie*; Verlag W. Kohlhammer: Stuttgart, Germany, 2018.
13. Liener, U.; Becker, C.; Rapp, K.; Raschke, M.; Kladny, B.; Wirtz, D. *Weissbuch Alterstraumatologie und Orthogeriatrie*; Verlag W. Kohlhammer: Stuttgart, Germany, 2021.
14. Varady, N.H.; Ameen, B.T.; Schwab, P.; Yeung, C.M.; Chen, A.F. Trends in the surgical treatment of pathological proximal femur fractures in the United States. *J. Surg. Oncol.* **2019**, *120*, 994–1007. [CrossRef] [PubMed]
15. Tsuda, Y.; Yasunaga, H.; Horiguchi, H.; Fushimi, K.; Kawano, H.; Tanaka, S. Complications and Postoperative Mortality Rate After Surgery for Pathological Femur Fracture Related to Bone Metastasis: Analysis of a Nationwide Database. *Ann. Surg. Oncol.* **2015**, *23*, 801–810. [CrossRef] [PubMed]
16. Varady, N.H.; Ameen, B.T.; Chen, A.F. Is Delayed Time to Surgery Associated with Increased Short-term Complications in Patients with Pathologic Hip Fractures? *Clin. Orthop. Relat. Res.* **2020**, *478*, 607–615. [CrossRef]
17. AUC—Akademie der Unfallchirurgie; Arbeitskreis AltersTraumaRegister DGU®. The geriatric trauma register of the DGU-current status, methods and publication guidelines. *Unfallchirurg* **2019**, *122*, 820–822.
18. Bücking, B.; Hartwig, E.; Nienaber, U.; Krause, U.; Friess, T.; Liener, U.; Hevia, M.; Bliemel, C.; Knobe, M.; AltersTraumaRegister DGU®. Results of the pilot phase of the Age Trauma Registry DGU®. *Unfallchirurg* **2017**, *120*, 619–624. [CrossRef]
19. Ho, D.; Imai, K.; King, G.; Stuart, E.A. MatchIt: Nonparametric Preprocessing for Parametric Causal Inference. *J. Stat. Softw.* **2011**, *42*, 1–28. [CrossRef]
20. Hansen, B.B.; Klopfer, S.O. Optimal Full Matching and Related Designs via Network Flows. *J. Comput. Graph. Stat.* **2006**, *15*, 609–627. [CrossRef]
21. McCusker, J.; Bellavance, F.; Cardin, S.; Trepanier, S.; Verdon, J.; Ardman, O.; McCusker, D.J.; Msc, S.T.; Msc, O.O.A. Detection of Older People at Increased Risk of Adverse Health Outcomes After an Emergency Visit: The ISAR Screening Tool. *J. Am. Geriatr. Soc.* **1999**, *47*, 1229–1237. [CrossRef]
22. Harvey, N.; Ahlmann, E.R.; Allison, D.C.; Wang, L.; Menendez, L.R. Endoprostheses Last Longer Than Intramedullary Devices in Proximal Femur Metastases. *Clin. Orthop. Relat. Res.* **2012**, *470*, 684–691. [CrossRef]
23. Steensma, M.; Boland, P.J.; Morris, C.D.; Athanasian, E.; Healey, J.H. Endoprosthetic Treatment is More Durable for Pathologic Proximal Femur Fractures. *Clin. Orthop. Relat. Res.* **2012**, *470*, 920–926. [CrossRef] [PubMed]
24. Houdek, M.T.; Wyles, C.C.; Labott, J.R.; Rose, P.S.; Taunton, M.J.; Sim, F.H. Durability of Hemiarthroplasty for Pathologic Proximal Femur Fractures. *J. Arthroplast.* **2017**, *32*, 3607–3610. [CrossRef] [PubMed]
25. Barahona, M.; Barrientos, C.; Cavada, G.; Brañes, J.; Martinez, Á.; Catalan, J. Survival analysis after hip fracture: Higher mortality than the general population and delayed surgery increases the risk at any time. *HIP Int.* **2020**, *30*, 54–58. [CrossRef] [PubMed]
26. Bliemel, C.; Rascher, K.; Knauf, T.; Hack, J.; Eschbach, D.; Aigner, R.; Oberkircher, L.; AltersTraumaRegister DGU®. Early Surgery Does Not Improve Outcomes for Patients with Periprosthetic Femoral Fractures—Results from the Registry for Geriatric Trauma of the German Trauma Society. *Medicina* **2021**, *57*, 517. [CrossRef]
27. Varady, N.H.; Ameen, B.T.; Hayden, B.L.; Yeung, C.M.; Schwab, P.-E.; Chen, A.F. Short-Term Morbidity and Mortality After Hemiarthroplasty and Total Hip Arthroplasty for Pathologic Proximal Femur Fractures. *J. Arthroplast.* **2019**, *34*, 2698–2703. [CrossRef] [PubMed]
28. Buecking, B.; Timmesfeld, N.; Riem, S.; Bliemel, C.; Hartwig, E.; Friess, T.; Liener, U.; Ruchholtz, S.; Eschbach, D. Early orthogeriatric treatment of trauma in the elderly: A systematic review and metaanalysis. *Dtsch Arztebl Int.* **2013**, *110*, 255–262.

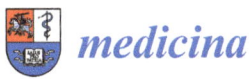

Article

COVID-19 Elderly Patients Treated for Proximal Femoral Fractures during the Second Wave of Pandemic in Italy and Iran: A Comparison between Two Countries

Riccardo Giorgino [1,*], Erfan Soroush [2], Sajjad Soroush [2], Sara Malakouti [2], Haniyeh Salari [2], Valeria Vismara [1], Filippo Migliorini [3], Riccardo Accetta [4] and Laura Mangiavini [4,5]

1. Residency Program in Orthopedics and Traumatology, University of Milan, 20122 Milan, Italy; valeria.vismara@unimi.it
2. Faculty of Medicine and Surgery, University of Milan, 20122 Milan, Italy; erfan.soroush@unimi.it (E.S.); sajjad.soroush@unimi.it (S.S.); sara.malakouti@unimi.it (S.M.); haniyeh.salari@unimi.it (H.S.)
3. Department of Orthopaedics, University Clinic Aachen, RWTH Aachen University Clinic, 52074 Aachen, Germany; migliorini.md@gmail.com
4. IRCCS Istituto Ortopedico Galeazzi, 20161 Milan, Italy; riccacc@gmail.com (R.A.); laura.mangiavini@unimi.it (L.M.)
5. Department of Biomedical Sciences for Health, University of Milan, 20161 Milan, Italy
* Correspondence: riccardo.giorgino@unimi.it; Tel.: +39-02-6621-4494

Citation: Giorgino, R.; Soroush, E.; Soroush, S.; Malakouti, S.; Salari, H.; Vismara, V.; Migliorini, F.; Accetta, R.; Mangiavini, L. COVID-19 Elderly Patients Treated for Proximal Femoral Fractures during the Second Wave of Pandemic in Italy and Iran: A Comparison between Two Countries. *Medicina* 2022, 58, 781. https://doi.org/10.3390/medicina58060781

Academic Editor: Carsten Schoeneberg

Received: 15 April 2022
Accepted: 6 June 2022
Published: 9 June 2022

Publisher's Note: MDPI stays neutral with regard to jurisdictional claims in published maps and institutional affiliations.

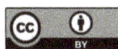

Copyright: © 2022 by the authors. Licensee MDPI, Basel, Switzerland. This article is an open access article distributed under the terms and conditions of the Creative Commons Attribution (CC BY) license (https://creativecommons.org/licenses/by/4.0/).

Abstract: *Background and objevtive*: The worldwide spread of SARS-CoV-2 has affected the various regions of the world differently. Italy and Iran have experienced a different adaptation to coexistence with the pandemic. Above all, fractures of the femur represent a large part of the necessary care for elderly patients. The aim of this study was to compare the treatment in Italy and Iran of COVID-19-positive patients suffering from proximal femur fractures in terms of characteristics, comorbidities, outcomes and complications. *Materials and Methods*: Medical records of COVID-19-positive patients with proximal femoral fractures treated at IRCCS Istituto Ortopedico Galeazzi in Milan (Italy) and at Salamat Farda and Parsa hospitals in the province of Tehran (Iran), in the time frame from 1 October 2020 to 16 January 2021, were analyzed and compared. *Results*: Records from 37 Italian patients and 33 Iranian patients were analyzed. The Italian group (mean age: 83.89 ± 1.60 years) was statistically older than the Iranian group (mean age: 75.18 ± 1.62 years) (p value = 0.0003). The mean number of transfusions for each patient in Italy was higher than the Iranian mean number (p value = 0.0062). The length of hospital stay in Italy was longer than in Iran (p value < 0.0001). Furthermore, laboratory values were different in the post-operative value of WBC and admission and post-operative values of CRP. *Conclusions*: The present study shows that differences were found between COVID-19-positive patients with proximal femoral fractures in these two countries. Further studies are required to validate these results and to better explain the reasons behind these differences.

Keywords: SARS-CoV-2; proximal femoral fractures; traumatology; clinical features; second wave; Italy; Iran

1. Introduction

The worldwide spread of severe acute respiratory syndrome coronavirus 2 (SARS-CoV-2) has affected the various regions of the world differently, with diverse modes of diffusion and saturation of the health system [1]. During the first SARS-Cov-2 wave, Italy was one of the most hit countries; meanwhile, even in Iran, the spread of COVID-19 led to a dramatic situation from the perspective of management of the medical assistance activity [2–4]. These two nations have experienced a different adaptation to coexistence with the pandemic, profoundly changing the daily life activities and medical practice [5–8] by setting limitations and restrictions and adapting assistance activities to cope with the emergency [9–11]. The second wave, on the other hand, found both countries prepared to face the health emergency, having already allowed the opportunity to set up assistance protocols and organize a hierarchical priority in medical-assistance activities [12,13]. In particular, with the regular reopening of social and work activities, some pathologies have returned to play an important role in the request for management by health facilities. Furthermore, the new welfare organizations had to consider as ordinary those patients affected by COVID-19, which in itself guarantees a notable picture of comorbidity and care difficulties. It is well known that fractures of the femur represent a large part of the necessary care for elderly patients [14,15] and have been a fundamental item in the organization of the new protocols [16]. In the evaluation of these fragile patients, different research groups tried to better understand how COVID-19 infection impacted the management, morbidity and mortality of such patients [17–20]. Nevertheless, a direct comparison between different countries is lacking. With these assumptions, it was of particular interest to compare how these elderly and complex patients were treated in two countries that have faced the second wave of the pandemic. The aim of this study was to compare patients' characteristics and treatment in Italy and Iran of COVID-19-positive elderly patients suffering from proximal femur fractures in terms of characteristics, comorbidities, outcomes and complications.

2. Materials and Methods

In this retrospective study, the medical records of COVID-19-positive patients with proximal femoral fractures treated at IRCCS Istituto Ortopedico Galeazzi in Milan (Italy) during the second wave of the pandemic, in the time frame from 1 October 2020 to 16 January 2021, were analyzed and compared with COVID-19-positive patients with proximal femoral fractures in the same timeframe treated at Salamat Farda and Parsa hospitals in the province of Tehran (Iran). Only COVID-19-positive patients were included in the study. Infection with SARS-COV-2 was detected in the majority of cases upon hospital arrival due to screening implemented by both the Italian and Iranian institutes with an RT-PCR test after nasopharyngeal swab. All patients underwent antithrombotic prophylaxis and were surgically treated. Data of each patient were collected from the medical records. Patients' characteristics (such as age, sex, comorbidities, diagnosis, laterality), treatment, length of hospital stay, complications, oxygen support, transfusions, discharge mode and laboratory values (hemoglobin, hematocrit, platelet count, C-reactive protein, white blood cells and creatinine) were evaluated. Laboratory values were collected in three stages: upon admission, at 3 to 5 days after surgery and at discharge. Complications were collected and grouped according to the physio-pathological sphere into the following: cardiovascular, metabolic, respiratory, oncological, nephrological, neuropsychiatric and other (gastrointestinal, immunological).

The analysis was performed using SPSS software version 26 (IBM SPSS Statistics, Chicago, IL, USA). Categorical variables (number of patients in each group, surgical treatment, oxygen support) in the two groups were described using counts and percentages, whereas mean and standard error were used to report continuous variables (age, number of transfusions, length of hospital stay). Binomial tests were used to compare the two groups according to classification of comorbidities. Laboratory values (hemoglobin, hematocrit, platelet count, CRP, WBC and creatinine) at three different time intervals were compared among the two groups using the unpaired Student's t-test to evaluate the normal data distribution. Significance was set at p value < 0.05.

3. Results

The COVID-19 Italian group was composed of 37 patients (10 males and 27 females), while the Iranian group was composed of 33 patients (10 males and 23 females). The Italian group was statistically older than the Iranian group, respectively, with a mean age of 83.89 ± 1.60 years vs. 75.18 ± 1.62 years (p value = 0.0003). All proximal femoral fractures were surgically treated. More precisely, in Italy, 1 total hip arthroplasty (THA), 10 bipolar hemiarthroplasties (BH) and 26 proximal femoral nails (PFN) were performed. In Iran, 5 patients were treated with THA, 15 with BH, 6 with PFN and 7 with dynamic hip screws

(DHS). In both groups, cardiovascular comorbidities were the most frequent. In Italy, 29 patients had cardiovascular comorbidities, 14 metabolic, 4 respiratory, 6 oncological, 2 nephrological, 8 neuropsychiatric, 2 other comorbidities, and 1 patient had none. In Iran, 17 patients had cardiovascular comorbidities, 15 metabolic, 4 respiratory, 1 oncological, 6 nephrological, 3 neuropsychiatric, 4 other comorbidities, and 2 patients had none. Upon admission, while only 18 patients in Italy (48.6%) were treated with oxygen support, all Iranian patients were treated with oxygen support (100%). The mean number of transfusions for each patient in Italy was 3.08 ± 0.50, and it emerged as statistically higher than the Iranian mean number of 2.12 ± 0.92 (p value = 0.0062). The length of hospital stay in Italy was longer than in Iran, with 13.24 ± 1.18 days vs. 4.27 ± 0.32 days (p value < 0.0001). All patients survived surgery in the early post-operative period. When focusing our attention on laboratory values (hemoglobin, hematocrit, platelet count, C-reactive protein, white blood cells and creatinine), comparisons of the two groups upon admission, 3/5 post-operative day and discharge are presented in Table 1.

Table 1. Comparison between laboratory values of COVID-19 Italian and Iranian groups upon admission, 3–5 post-operative day and discharge.

Lab Values	Admission		3–5 Postoperative Day		Discharge	
	Italy	Iran	Italy	Iran	Italy	Iran
Hemoglobin (g/dL)	11.90 ± 035	12.24 ± 0.31	10.24 ± 0.22	10.61 ± 0.25	11.31 ± 0.71	10.01 ± 0.27
Hematocrit (%)	36.99 ± 1.02	35.88 ± 1.02	31.79 ± 0.68	31.30 ± 0.76	33.75 ± 0.81	30.31 ± 0.88
Platelet count (10³/μL)	265.41 ± 19.48	269.45 ± 18.64	276.84 ± 16.44	249.57 ± 16.56	321.12 ± 31.84	285.07 ± 18.94
CRP (mg/L)	5.40 ± 0.87	2.50 ± 0.19	7.89 ± 1.28	3.41 ± 0.24	4.79 ± 0.97	3.21 ± 0.18
WBC (10³/μL)	10.72 ± 1.11	11.73 ± 1.09	11.50 ± 1.46	9.79 ± 0.62	10.46 ± 0.93	10.89 ± 0.59
Creatinine (mg/dL)	0.96 ± 0.06	1.02 ± 0.07	1.22 ± 0.30	1.04 ± 0.09	0.83 ± 0.07	0.96 ± 0.09

The post-operative value of white blood cells in the Italian group was statistically higher than in the Iranian sample, with a mean value of 11.50 ± 1.46 vs. 9.79 ± 0.62 (p value = 0.0288) (Figure 1).

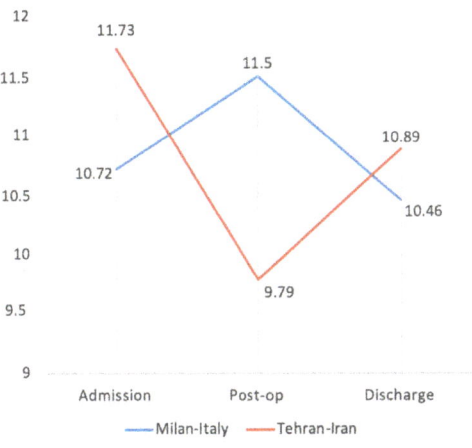

Figure 1. Trend of white blood cells (WBC) in COVID-19 Italian and Iranian groups.

The admission value of CRP in the Italian group was statistically higher than in the Iranian one, with a mean value of 5.40 ± 0.87 vs. 2.50 ± 0.19 (p value = 0.0025). The same statistical difference is still present at the post-operative values (7.89 ± 1.28 vs. 3.41 ± 0.24 (p value = 0.0014), as can be seen in Figure 2.

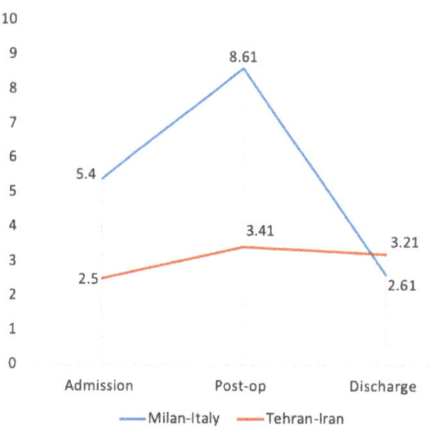

Figure 2. Trend of C-reactive protein (CRP) in COVID-19 Italian and Iranian groups.

4. Discussion

The main clinical relevance of the present study resides in the analysis of the differences in the management of important pathologies in the assistance activity of orthopedics, such as proximal femur fractures, between two different countries during a pandemic never seen before. According to the main findings of this study, many differences were found through the analysis of these two groups. The Italian group was statistically older than the Iranian group, with a longer length of hospital stay and a higher mean number of transfusions for each patient in Italy. Furthermore, concerning laboratory indices, WBC post-operative values and both CRP admission and post-operative values were significantly different. As mentioned above, the length of hospital stay in Italy was longer than in Iran, with 13.24 ± 1.18 days vs. 4.27 ± 0.32 days (p value < 0.0001). In particular, it should be emphasized that the patients of the Iranian group were hospitalized in private facilities, and therefore, the length of the hospital stay was undoubtedly influenced by the sudden transfer to physiotherapy wards for several reasons, including economic ones. Moreover, most rehabilitative structures in Italy, to avoid the spread of the SARS-COV-2 infection, avoid taking patients in until a negative test is available, thereby increasing the hospital length of stay. Nevertheless, encouraging evidence in the literature suggests that an enhanced recovery after surgery (ERAS) protocol can benefit patients with hip fractures [21], but undoubtedly, in the case of a patient suffering from COVID-19, the matter becomes more complicated by having to interface with further timelines linked to specific anti-COVID protocols. This is an important aspect, as we have already previously described how our hospital was able to improve some parameters of hospital clinical efficiency during the first wave of the pandemic. Indeed, in the study of Brayda-Bruno et al., the time frames from diagnosis to surgery and from diagnosis to discharge were analyzed, reporting a reduction in diagnosis–discharge time [22]. The increased length of stay of the Italian patients could even be related to the higher age in the Italian group, as already underlined in the literature, where older age is correlated with a longer length of stay [23,24]. However, other studies did not report a correlation between advanced age in patients with femoral fractures and a prolonged hospital stay [25,26].

Regarding the laboratory data shown in the table, there are some considerations to emphasize. In our results, we found that post-operative value of WBC was statistically higher in the Italian group compared to the Iranian patients. It has been reported in the literature that among trauma patients, higher WBC values were detected in patients with major lesions rather than in patients with minor lesions, but both were within the normal range [27]. These data should be integrated with what emerges from recent studies on COVID-19 patients, where it was described that WBC count in COVID-19 patients is normal or slightly reduced in the early stages and that these values may change as the disease progresses [28]. Furthermore, recent studies suggest that various parameters, including WBC, could predict critical disease progression [29]. Another result that emerged from our study was the finding of higher values of CRP in the Italian group upon admission and post-operative time. For all COVID-19 patients, we should consider a high level of inflammation due to the nature of COVID-19 disease [30–32]. Indeed, in the study of Puzzitiello et al., it is reported how these patients with orthopedic trauma injuries may have an amplified response to the traumatic insult because of their baseline hyperinflammatory and hypercoagulable states [33]. The same findings were confirmed by Bayrak et al., where inflammatory parameters, including CRP, were higher in COVID-19-positive patients with femoral fractures [34]. Our results are adequately framed within the literature findings; however, further studies should be conducted to explain the reason for the laboratory differences between the patients of the two countries.

This study presents several limitations. First of all, it is a case series. Second, the collection of clinical documentation was conducted in two different countries in line with the primary objective of this work in the study of differences. However, this collection of data had to face different pre-operative, surgical and post-operative treatment protocols, as already illustrated above. In this respect, it is not easy to compare the pre-operative preparation and surgical technique of different surgeons from two different countries. Third, there is still little literature about the differences of COVID-19-positive patients among different countries, and future studies should investigate any differences and points in common in order to establish the best possible treatment throughout the duration of the medical intervention. Furthermore, possibly, further studies should increase the sample size, which, in the present work, is already important, considering the sampling of patients. Another limitation is scarce information about the COVID-19 infection of these patients (onset of infection, severity, quantity of oxygen support needed, relationship with patient outcomes). Due to the above-mentioned difficulties in collecting data, some records about the onset of the viral infection and the symptoms are lacking. In particular, we do not know if the traumatic event might have been directly related to the COVID-19 infection (i.e., due to muscular weakness); it is also highly possible that our patients were hospitalized and treated in different stages of the viral infection, thus affecting the evaluated outcomes. Finally, another important aspect that constitutes a limitation resides in the follow-up of these patients, which is limited to the few days of hospital stay in the post-operative period. Further studies should be able to evaluate the survival of COVID-19 patients surgically treated precisely in order to perhaps be able to draw up international guidelines.

5. Conclusions

The present study shows that some differences were found between COVID-19-positive patients with proximal femoral fractures in Italy and Iran in terms of mean age, length of hospital stay, number of transfusions, WBC count and CRP values. Further studies are required to validate these results, to better explain the reasons behind these differences and to establish the best treatment throughout the duration of the medical intervention.

Author Contributions: Conceptualization, R.G. and L.M.; methodology, L.M.; software, E.S., S.S., S.M. and H.S.; validation, R.G., L.M. and F.M.; formal analysis, L.M.; investigation, R.G., V.V., E.S., S.S., S.M., H.S. and R.A.; writing—original draft preparation, R.G.; writing—review and editing, L.M.; supervision, L.M. and R.A. All authors have read and agreed to the published version of the manuscript.

Funding: This research received no external funding.

Institutional Review Board Statement: The study was conducted according to the guidelines of the Declaration of Helsinki. Ethical review and approval were waived for this study due to sensitive and personal data being treated anonymously.

Informed Consent Statement: Patient consent was waived due to sensitive and personal data being treated anonymously.

Data Availability Statement: Data supporting the reported results can be found in database generated during the study.

Acknowledgments: The authors wish to thank Zabihollah Hassanzade and Sara Soroush for their contribution to the paper.

Conflicts of Interest: The authors declare no conflict of interest.

References

1. Huang, C.; Wang, Y.; Li, X.; Ren, L.; Zhao, J.; Hu, Y.; Zhang, L.; Yu, Z.; Fang, M.; Yu, T.; et al. Clinical features of patients infected with 2019 novel coronavirus in Wuhan, China. *Lancet* **2020**, *395*, 497–506. [CrossRef]
2. Zagra, L.; Faraldi, M.; Pregliasco, F.; Vinci, A.; Lombardi, G.; Ottaiano, I.; Accetta, R.; Perazzo, P.; D'Apolito, R. Changes of clinical activities in an orthopaedic institute in North Italy during the spread of COVID-19 pandemic: A seven-week observational analysis. *Int. Orthop.* **2020**, *44*, 1591–1598. [CrossRef] [PubMed]
3. Ambrosio, L.; Vadalà, G.; Russo, F.; Papalia, R.; Denaro, V. The role of the orthopaedic surgeon in the COVID-19 era: Cautions and perspectives. *J. Exp. Orthop.* **2020**, *7*, 35. [CrossRef] [PubMed]
4. Perazzo, P.; Giorgino, R.; Briguglio, M.; Zuffada, M.; Accetta, R.; Mangiavini, L.; Peretti, G.M. From Standard to Escalated Anticoagulant Prophylaxis in Fractured Older Adults With SARS-CoV-2 Undergoing Accelerated Orthopedic Surgery. *Front. Med.* **2020**, *7*, 566770. [CrossRef]
5. Giorgino, R.; Maggioni, D.M.; Viganò, M.; Verdoni, F.; Pandini, E.; Balbino, C.; Manta, N.; D'Anchise, R.; Mangiavini, L. Knee Pathology before and after SARS-CoV-2 Pandemic: An Analysis of 1139 Patients. *Healthcare* **2021**, *9*, 1311. [CrossRef]
6. Albano, D.; Bruno, A.; Bruno, F.; Calandri, M.; Caruso, D.; Clemente, A.; Coppolino, P.; Cozzi, D.; De Robertis, R.; Gentili, F.; et al. Impact of coronavirus disease 2019 (COVID-19) emergency on Italian radiologists: A national survey. *Eur. Radiol.* **2020**, *30*, 6635–6644. [CrossRef]
7. Tagliafico, A.S.; Albano, D.; Torri, L.; Messina, C.; Gitto, S.; Bruno, F.; Barileg, A.; Giovagnonih, A.; Mielei, V.; Grassi, R.; et al. Impact of coronavirus disease 2019 (COVID-19) outbreak on radiology research: An Italian survey. *Clin. Imaging* **2021**, *76*, 144–148. [CrossRef]
8. Catellani, F.; Coscione, A.; D'Ambrosi, R.; Usai, L.; Roscitano, C.; Fiorentino, G. Treatment of Proximal Femoral Fragility Fractures in Patients with COVID-19 During the SARS-CoV-2 Outbreak in Northern Italy. *J. Bone Joint Surg. Am.* **2020**, *102*, e58. [CrossRef]
9. Morelli, I.; Luceri, F.; Giorgino, R.; Accetta, R.; Perazzo, P.; Mangiavini, L.; Maffulli, N.; Peretti, G.M. COVID-19: Not a contraindication for surgery in patients with proximal femur fragility fractures. *J. Orthop. Surg. Res.* **2020**, *15*, 285. [CrossRef]
10. Briguglio, M.; Giorgino, R.; Dell'Osso, B.; Cesari, M.; Porta, M.; Lattanzio, F.; Banfi, G.; Peretti, G.M. Consequences for the Elderly After COVID-19 Isolation: FEaR (Frail Elderly amid Restrictions). *Front. Psychol.* **2020**, *11*, 565052. [CrossRef]
11. Ahmadi, Z.H.; Mousavizadeh, M.; Nikpajouh, A.; Bahsir, M.; Hosseini, S. COVID-19: A perspective from Iran. *J. Card. Surg.* **2021**, *36*, 1672–1676. [CrossRef] [PubMed]
12. D'Ambrosi, R.; Biazzo, A.; Masia, F.; Izzo, V.; Confalonieri, N.; Ursino, N.; Verde, F. Guidelines for Resuming Elective Hip and Knee Surgical Activity Following the COVID-19 Pandemic: An Italian Perspective. *HSS J.* **2020**, *16*, 71–76. [CrossRef] [PubMed]
13. Cacciapaglia, G.; Cot, C.; Sannino, F. Second wave COVID-19 pandemics in Europe: A temporal playbook. *Sci. Rep.* **2020**, *10*, 15514. [CrossRef] [PubMed]
14. Migliorini, F.; Giorgino, R.; Hildebrand, F.; Spiezia, F.; Peretti, G.M.; Alessandri-Bonetti, M.; Eschweiler, J.; Maffulli, N. Fragility Fractures: Risk Factors and Management in the Elderly. *Medicina* **2021**, *57*, 1119. [CrossRef]
15. Kanis, J.A.; Odén, A.; McCloskey, E.V.; Johansson, H.; Wahl, D.A.; Cooper, C. A systematic review of hip fracture incidence and probability of fracture worldwide. *Osteoporos. Int.* **2012**, *23*, 2239–2256. [CrossRef]
16. Hall, A.J.; Clement, N.D.; Farrow, L.; MacLullich, A.M.J.; Dall, G.F.; Scott, C.E.H.; Jenkins, P.J.; White, T.O.; Duckworth, A.D. IMPACT-Scot report on COVID-19 and hip fractures. *Bone Joint J.* **2020**, *102*, 1219–1228. [CrossRef]
17. Pass, B.; Vajna, E.; Knauf, T.; Rascher, K.; Aigner, R.; Eschbach, D.; Lendemans, S.; Knobe, M.; Schoeneberg, C.; the Registry for Geriatric Trauma (ATR-DGU). COVID-19 and Proximal Femur Fracture in Older Adults-A Lethal Combination? An Analysis of the Registry for Geriatric Trauma (ATR-DGU). *J. Am. Med. Dir. Assoc.* **2021**, *23*, 576–580. [CrossRef]
18. Ward, A.E.; Tadross, D.; Wells, F.; Majkowski, L.; Naveed, U.; Jeyapalan, R.; Partridge, D.G.; Madan, S.; Blundell, C.M. The impact of COVID-19 on morbidity and mortality in neck of femur fracture patients: A prospective case-control cohort study. *Bone Jt. Open* **2020**, *1*, 669–675. [CrossRef]
19. Wignall, A.; Giannoudis, V.; De, C.; Jimenez, A.; Sturdee, S.; Nisar, S.; Pandit, H.; Gulati, A.; Palan, J. The impact of COVID-19 on the management and outcomes of patients with proximal femoral fractures: A multi-centre study of 580 patients. *J. Orthop. Surg. Res.* **2021**, *16*, 155. [CrossRef]

20. COVIDSurg Collaborative. Outcomes after perioperative SARS-CoV-2 infection in patients with proximal femoral fractures: An international cohort study. *BMJ Open* **2021**, *11*, e050830. [CrossRef]
21. Liu, S.-Y.; Li, C.; Zhang, P.-X. Enhanced recovery after surgery for hip fractures: A systematic review and meta-analysis. *Perioper. Med.* **2021**, *10*, 31. [CrossRef] [PubMed]
22. Brayda-Bruno, M.; Giorgino, R.; Gallazzi, E.; Morelli, I.; Manfroni, F.; Briguglio, M.; Accetta, R.; Mangiavini, L.; Peretti, G.M. How SARS-CoV-2 Pandemic Changed Traumatology and Hospital Setting: An Analysis of 498 Fractured Patients. *J. Clin. Med.* **2021**, *10*, 2585. [CrossRef] [PubMed]
23. Muhm, M.; Walendowski, M.; Danko, T.; Weiss, C.; Ruffing, T.; Winkler, H. Factors influencing course of hospitalization in patients with hip fractures: Complications, length of stay and hospital mortality. *Z. Gerontol. Geriatr.* **2015**, *48*, 339–345. [CrossRef] [PubMed]
24. Muhm, M.; Walendowski, M.; Danko, T.; Weiss, C.; Ruffing, T.; Winkler, H. Length of hospital stay for patients with proximal femoral fractures: Influencing factors. *Unfallchirurg* **2016**, *119*, 560–569. [CrossRef] [PubMed]
25. Eschbach, D.-A.; Oberkircher, L.; Bliemel, C.; Mohr, J.; Ruchholtz, S.; Buecking, B. Increased age is not associated with higher incidence of complications, longer stay in acute care hospital and in hospital mortality in geriatric hip fracture patients. *Maturitas* **2013**, *74*, 185–189. [CrossRef] [PubMed]
26. Lott, A.; Belayneh, R.; Haglin, J.; Konda, S.R.; Egol, K.A. Age Alone Does Not Predict Complications, Length of Stay, and Cost for Patients Older Than 90 Years with Hip Fractures. *Orthopedics* **2019**, *42*, e51–e55. [CrossRef]
27. Paladino, L.; Subramanian, R.A.; Bonilla, E.; Sinert, R.H. Leukocytosis as prognostic indicator of major injury. *West J. Emerg. Med.* **2010**, *11*, 450–455.
28. Karimi Shahri, M.; Niazkar, H.R.; Rad, F. COVID-19 and hematology findings based on the current evidences: A puzzle with many missing pieces. *Int. J. Lab. Hematol.* **2021**, *43*, 160–168. [CrossRef]
29. Henry, B.M.; de Oliveira, M.H.S.; Benoit, S.; Plebani, M.; Lippi, G. Hematologic, biochemical and immune biomarker abnormalities associated with severe illness and mortality in coronavirus disease 2019 (COVID-19): A meta-analysis. *Clin. Chem. Lab. Med.* **2020**, *58*, 1021–1028. [CrossRef]
30. Leisman, D.E.; Deutschman, C.S.; Legrand, M. Facing COVID-19 in the ICU: Vascular dysfunction, thrombosis, and dysregulated inflammation. *Intensive Care Med.* **2020**, *46*, 1105–1108. [CrossRef]
31. Briguglio, M.; Porta, M.; Zuffada, F.; Bona, A.R.; Crespi, T.; Pino, F.; Perazzo, P.; Mazzocchi, M.; Giorgino, R.; De Angelis, G.; et al. SARS-CoV-2 Aiming for the Heart: A Multicenter Italian Perspective About Cardiovascular Issues in COVID-19. *Front. Physiol.* **2020**, *11*, 571367. [CrossRef]
32. Migliorini, F.; Torsiello, E.; Spiezia, F.; Oliva, F.; Tingart, M.; Maffulli, N. Association between HLA genotypes and COVID-19 susceptibility, severity and progression: A comprehensive review of the literature. *Eur. J. Med. Res.* **2021**, *26*, 84. [CrossRef] [PubMed]
33. Puzzitiello, R.N.; Pagani, N.R.; Moverman, M.A.; Moon, A.S.; Menendez, M.E.; Ryan, S.P. Inflammatory and Coagulative Considerations for the Management of Orthopaedic Trauma Patients With COVID-19: A Review of the Current Evidence and Our Surgical Experience. *J. Orthop. Trauma* **2020**, *34*, 389–394. [CrossRef] [PubMed]
34. Bayrak, A.; Duramaz, A.; Çakmur, B.B.; Kural, C.; Basaran, S.H.; Erçin, E.; Kural, A.; Ursavaş, H.T. The effect of COVID-19 positivity on inflammatory parameters and thirty day mortality rates in patients over sixty five years of age with surgically treated intertrochanteric fractures. *Int. Orthop.* **2021**, *45*, 3025–3031. [CrossRef] [PubMed]

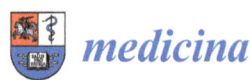

Article

Comparing Perioperative Outcome Measures of the Dynamic Hip Screw and the Femoral Neck System

Marcel Niemann [1,2,*], Karl F. Braun [1,3], Sufian S. Ahmad [1,4], Ulrich Stöckle [1], Sven Märdian [1] and Frank Graef [1]

1. Center for Musculoskeletal Surgery, Charité—Universitätsmedizin Berlin, Corporate Member of Freie Universität Berlin, Humboldt-Universität zu Berlin, Berlin Institute of Health, 13353 Berlin, Germany; karl.braun@charite.de (K.F.B.); sufian@ahmadortho.com (S.S.A.); ulrich.stoeckle@charite.de (U.S.); sven.maerdian@charite.de (S.M.); frank.graef@charite.de (F.G.)
2. Julius Wolff Institute for Biomechanics and Musculoskeletal Regeneration, Charité—Universitätsmedizin Berlin, 13353 Berlin, Germany
3. Department of Trauma Surgery, University Hospital Rechts der Isar, Technical University of Munich, 81675 Munich, Germany
4. Department of Orthopedic Surgery, Hannover Medical School, 30625 Hannover, Germany
* Correspondence: marcel.niemann@charite.de; Tel.: +49-30-450-652-356; Fax: +49-30-450-552-901

Abstract: *Background and Objective*: Various fixation devices and surgical techniques are available for the management of proximal femur fractures. Recently, the femoral neck system (FNS) was introduced, and was promoted on the basis of less invasiveness, shorter operating time, and less fluoroscopy time compared to previous systems. The aim of this study was to compare two systems for the internal fixation of femoral neck fractures (FNF), namely the dynamic hip screw (DHS) with an anti-rotation screw (ARS) and an FNS. The outcome measures included operating room time (ORT), dose–area product (DAP), length of stay (LOS), perioperative changes in haemoglobin concentrations, and transfusion rate. *Materials and Methods*: A retrospective single-centre study was conducted. Patients treated for FNF between 1 January 2020 and 30 September 2021 were included, provided that they had undergone closed reduction and internal fixation. We measured the centrum-collum-diaphyseal (CCD) and the Pauwels angle preoperatively and one week postoperatively. *Results*: In total, 31 patients (16 females), with a mean age of 62.81 ± 15.05 years, were included. Fracture complexity assessed by the Pauwels and Garden classification did not differ between groups preoperatively. Nonetheless, the ORT (54 ± 26.1 min vs. 91.68 ± 23.96 min, $p < 0.01$) and DAP (721 ± 270.6 cGycm^2 vs. 1604 ± 1178 cGycm^2, $p = 0.03$) were significantly lower in the FNS group. The pre- and postoperative CCD and Pauwels angles did not differ statistically between groups. Perioperative haemoglobin concentration changes (−1.77 ± 1.19 g/dl vs. −1.74 ± 1.37 g/dl) and LOS (8 ± 5.27 days vs. 7.35 ± 3.43 days) were not statistically different. *Conclusions*: In this cohort, the ORT and DAP were almost halved in the patient group treated with FNS. This may confer a reduction in secondary risks related to surgery.

Keywords: dynamic hip screw; femoral neck system; femoral neck fracture; individual medicine; minimal-invasive surgery; multiple trauma; geriatrics

Citation: Niemann, M.; Braun, K.F.; Ahmad, S.S.; Stöckle, U.; Märdian, S.; Graef, F. Comparing Perioperative Outcome Measures of the Dynamic Hip Screw and the Femoral Neck System. *Medicina* **2022**, *58*, 352. https://doi.org/10.3390/medicina58030352

Academic Editor: Carsten Schoeneberg

Received: 8 February 2022
Accepted: 24 February 2022
Published: 26 February 2022

Publisher's Note: MDPI stays neutral with regard to jurisdictional claims in published maps and institutional affiliations.

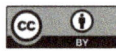

Copyright: © 2022 by the authors. Licensee MDPI, Basel, Switzerland. This article is an open access article distributed under the terms and conditions of the Creative Commons Attribution (CC BY) license (https://creativecommons.org/licenses/by/4.0/).

1. Introduction

Femoral neck fractures (FNF) have an enormous socioeconomic impact on modern society. The total number of hip fractures is expected to increase from 1.26 million in 1990 to 21.3 million by 2050 [1]. These fractures have been reported to negatively impact patients' functional status, quality of life, and independence [2]. Furthermore, fractures close to the hip are strongly associated with a pronounced risk of cardiovascular complications and mortality [3].

Several authors have worked on standardised treatment concept that take into account the fracture location, fracture classification, and patients' individual risk factors [4,5].

However, these concepts remain highly heterogeneous, especially regarding the indication for osteosynthetic reconstruction or replacement with a hemi- or total hip arthroplasty. Reconstruction is reserved for cases in which the perfusion of the femoral head is presumably not compromised. Therefore, broadly accepted fracture classification systems, such as the Pauwels [6] or Garden classification [7], help clinicians through the decision-making process. Accordingly, Pauwels type I and II and Garden type I and II fractures usually qualify for reconstruction.

Various implants for the reconstruction of an FNF are currently available. The dynamic hip screw (DHS) is the most commonly used system (Figure 1). When considering the implantation of a DHS, an additional anti-rotational screw (ARS) should explicitly be used in FNF to increase rotational stability. This combination has been associated with significantly improved traction and compression distribution on fractures [8], potentially facilitating a healing outcome. However, a recent meta-analysis observed no superiority regarding mortality, fracture consolidation rate, and revision rate when comparing the DHS to cannulated screws [9].

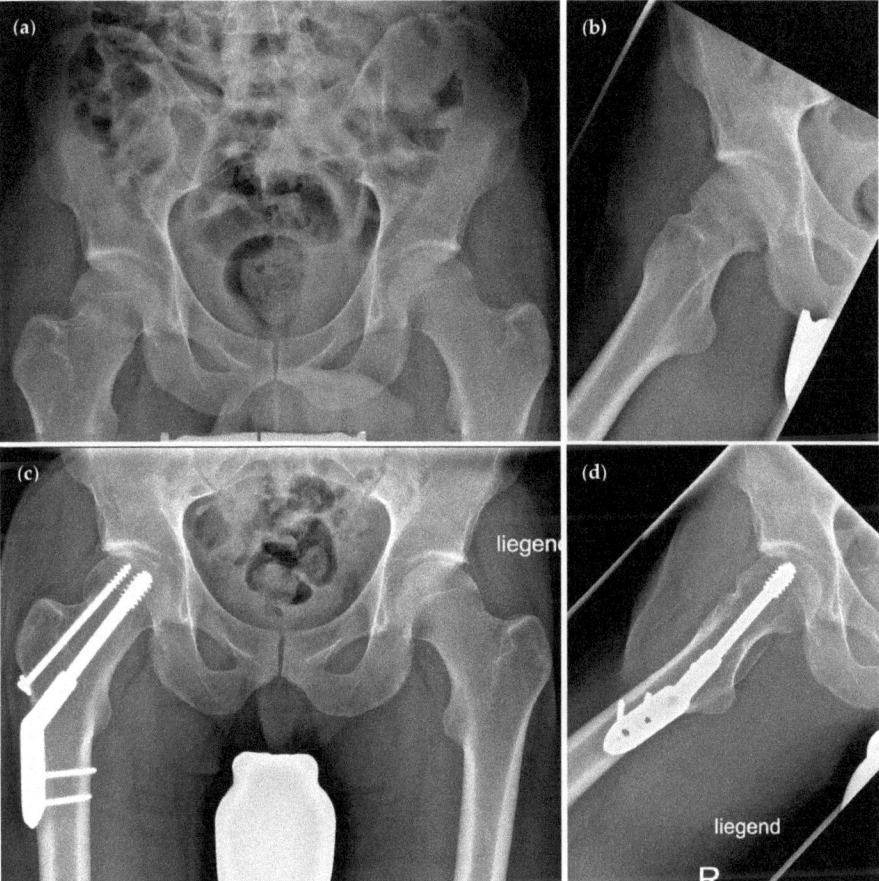

Figure 1. Radiographic visualisation of the dynamic hip screw (DHS) with anti-rotational screw (ARS). (**a**,**b**) Preoperative radiographs of a Garden type II/Pauwels type II femoral neck fracture. (**c**,**d**) Postoperative radiographs after osteosynthesis using a DHS with ARS.

Recently, a new and innovative reconstruction system was introduced: the femoral neck system (FNS) (DePuy Synthes, Raynham, MA, USA) (Figure 2) [10–12]. This system is exclusively designed to stabilise FNF. It allows for dynamic fixation of the femoral neck, rotational stability through a screw-in-screw concept, and increased strength at the shaft due to a locking screw. Thereby, it combines the biomechanical advantages of different well-known osteosynthesis principles. Furthermore, the FNS can be applied percutaneously while maintaining the beneficial characteristics of the DHS. Biomechanical studies have shown that the FNS is as a valid alternative to the DHS with ARS and is superior to cannulated screws for the management of Pauwels type III fractures [13]. Recent clinical studies have shown that reconstructions using the FNS lead to satisfactory perioperative and clinical outcome measures [14–18]. To date, only one group of authors has compared the FNS with the DHS for Garden type I and II fractures in elderly patients [17]. They observed a shorter operating room time (ORT) in the FNS group, but there were no differences in the transfusion rate, local complications, length of stay (LOS), or mortality between groups. However, only including elderly patients and Garden type I and II fractures may impair study data quality and limit the implications for other clinicians.

Therefore, this study aimed to compare all patients that were stabilised using either a DHS with ARS or FNS at our institution. Particular emphasis was given to the ORT, which was our primary outcome measure. Secondary outcome measures were dose–area product (DAP), LOS, change in haemoglobin concentrations, and transfusion rate.

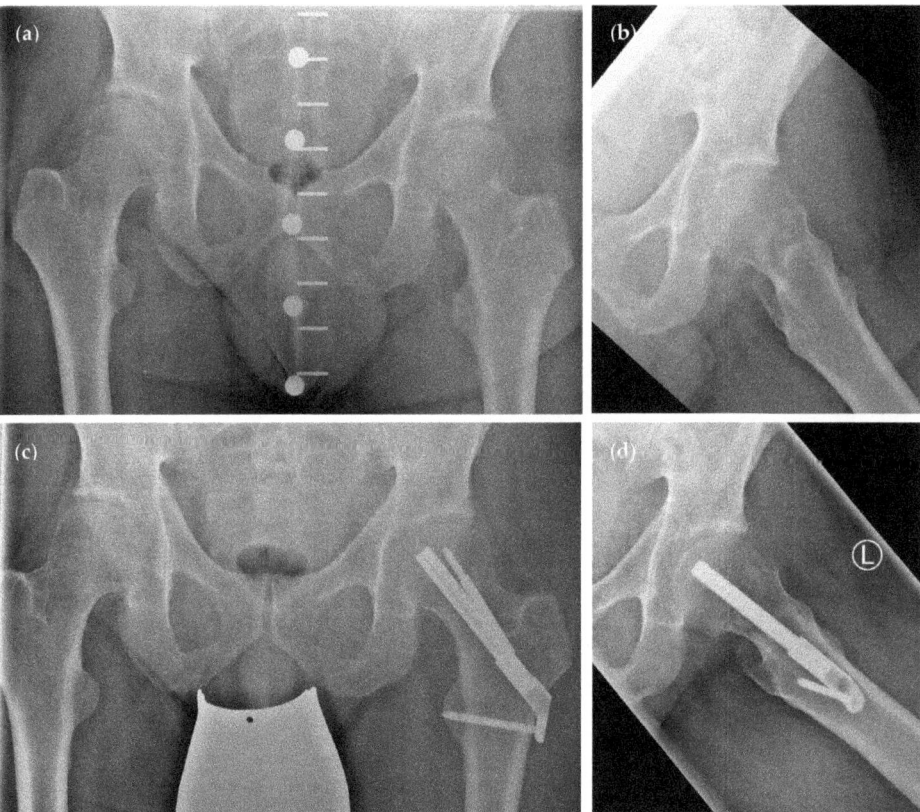

Figure 2. Radiographic visualisation of the femoral neck system (FNS). (**a**,**b**) Preoperative radiographs of a Garden type II/Pauwels type II femoral neck fracture. (**c**,**d**) Postoperative radiographs after osteosynthesis using the FNS.

2. Methods

We conducted a retrospective study examining all FNF patients being treated at our level 1 trauma centre between January 2020 and September 2021. Approval of the local institutional review board (application number EA4/141/21) was obtained before initiation of the study. Patient data (age, gender, the American Society of Anesthesiologists [ASA] physical status classification system, Charlson Comorbidity Index (CCI) [19], trauma mechanism, fracture type according to Pauwels and Garden, LOS, and complications following surgery) were extracted from the electronic medical data system, SAP (SAP ERP 6.0 EHP4, SAP AG, Walldorf, Germany). Furthermore, perioperative data were noted including time to surgery (TTS) (including patient positioning and closed fracture reduction), ORT, DAP, transfusion rate, perioperative volume therapy, and haemoglobin concentrations prior to and following surgery.

We assessed Pauwels and centrum–collum–diaphyseal (CCD) angles in pre- and postoperative plain anterior–posterior radiographs of the pelvis using MERLIN Diagnostic Workcenter (MERLIN Diagnostic Workcenter for Microsoft Windows, Version 5.8.1, Phönix-PACS GmbH, Freiburg im Breisgau, Germany). This is displayed in Figure 3.

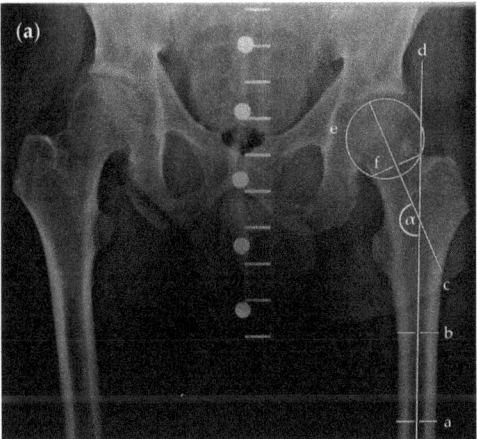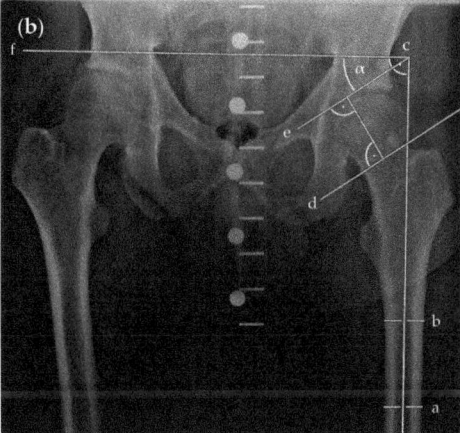

Figure 3. Radiographic visualisation of angle measurements in plain anterior–posterior radiographs of the pelvis. In (**a**), CCD angle (α) is measured between the longitudinal femoral shaft axis (d), determined by two bisections of the shaft (a, b), and the femoral neck axis (c), determined by the centre of the femoral head (centre of [e]) and its overlap with the femoral neck (f). In (**b**), fracture angle according to Pauwels classification (α) is measured between the fracture line (d or e) and the horizontal (f), which was perpendicular to the longitudinal femoral shaft axis (c), determined by two bisections of the shaft (a, b). Abbreviations: CCD, centrum–collum–diaphyseal.

Statistical analysis was performed using GraphPad Prism (GraphPad Prism 9 for macOS, Version 9.3.1 [350], GraphPad Holdings, LLC, San Diego, CA, USA). Data distribution was tested using histograms and Q–Q plots. The Mann–Whitney U test was used for discrete and continuous variables and Fisher's exact test was used for categorical variables. We performed outlier detection using the ROUT method with Q = 0.1% [20]. Unless otherwise stated, discrete and continuous variables are represented as the mean ± SD (95% CI), and categorical variables are presented as frequencies (%). All p-values are two tailed, and p-values < 0.05 were considered statistically significant.

3. Results

3.1. Demographics

Between January 2020 and September 2021, 31 patients (16 female) were operated on due to an FNF. Of these, 19 patients received a DHS with ARS and 12 patients received an FNS. In each group, two patients received an in situ fixation as the smallest possible intervention due to their individual perioperative risk constellations.

The mean age of the cohort was 62.81 ± 15.05 years (95% CI 57.28–68.33). Twenty-three patients (74.19%) had a low impact trauma (fall from standing height), four patients (12.9%) had a bicycle accident, two patients (6.45%) had a motorised scooter accident, one patient (3.23%) had an inline skate accident, and one patient (3.23%) had a car accident. A detailed overview of the study cohort is given in Table 1. We did not detect any significant differences between groups regarding the baseline characteristics. Especially, pre- and postoperative Pauwels classification and CCD angles did not differ between groups.

3.2. Outcome Measures

The ORT significantly differed (U = 24.5, p < 0.01) between the DHS group (91.68 ± 23.96 min, 95% CI 80.14–103.23) and the FNS group (54 ± 26.1 min, 95% CI 37.42–70.58). No outliers were detected.

The DAP was 1604.19 ± 1178.16 cGycm^2 (95% CI 1036.34–2172.04) in the DHS group and 721 ± 270.65 cGycm^2 (95% CI 527.39–914.61) in the FNS group. Analysis revealed a significant difference between groups (U = 47, p = 0.03). One outlier was identified in the FNS group (DAP of 5407.25 cGycm^2) and was excluded prior to analysis.

Haemoglobin concentration changes were highly comparable between the DHS group (−1.74 ± 1.37 mg/dL, 95% CI −2.42−−1.06) and the FNS group (−1.77 ± 1.19 mg/dL, 95% CI −2.52−−1.01) (U = 104.5, p = 0.89). No outliers were detected.

The LOS was 7.35 ± 3.43 days (95% CI 5.59–9.12) in the DHS group and 8 ± 5.27 days (95% CI 4.65–11.35) in the FNS group. The differences between groups were not significant (U = 100, p = 0.94). Two outliers were identified in the DHS group (LOS of 26 and 43 days) and were excluded prior to analysis.

Figure 4 shows the assessed outcome measures.

Table 1. Overview of the study cohort.

		DHS (n = 19)	FNS (n = 12)	Statistics
	Age (years)	60.47 ± 17 (95% CI 52.28–68.67)	66.5 ± 10.98 (95% CI 59.52–73.48)	p = 0.34
Gender	Female (% of group)	10 (52.63%)	6 (50%)	p = 1
	Male (% of group)	9 (47.37%)	6 (50%)	
	ASA	2.32 ± 0.75 (95% CI 1.96–2.68)	2.42 ± 0.67 (95% CI 1.99–2.84)	p = 0.81
	CCI	3.16 ± 3.39 (95% CI 1.53–4.79)	4.42 ± 3.7 (95% CI 2.06–6.77)	p = 0.38
	Preoperative Pauwels angle (°)	50.93 ± 14.07 (95% CI 44.15–57.71)	47.66 ± 14.44 (95% CI 38.49–56.83)	p = 0.41
	Postoperative Pauwels angle (°)	46.74 ± 7.71 (95% CI 43.03–50.46)	43.34 ± 7.93 (95% CI 38.3–48.38)	p = 0.22
	Preoperative CCD angle (°)	129.5 ± 16.21 (95% CI 121.7–137.3)	130.8 ± 13.25 (95% CI 122.4–139.2)	p = 0.8
	Postoperative CCD angle (°)	135.9 ± 7.27 (95% CI 132.4–139.4)	136 ± 5.24 (95% CI 132.7–139.4)	p = 0.85

Table 1. *Cont.*

		DHS (n = 19)	FNS (n = 12)	Statistics
Pauwels classification	Type I (% of group)	1 (5.26%)	1 (8.33%)	$p = 0.72$ *
	Type II (% of group)	10 (52.63%)	7 (58.33%)	
	Type III (% of group)	8 (42.11%)	4 (33.33%)	
Garden classification	Type I (% of group)	2 (10.53%)	1 (8.33%)	$p = 0.45$ **
	Type II (% of group)	9 (47.37%)	8 (66.67%)	
	Type III (% of group)	4 (21.05%)	2 (16.67%)	
	Type IV (% of group)	4 (21.05%)	1 (8.33%)	
TTS (min)		44.74 ± 10.66 (95% CI 39.6–49.87)	48.83 ± 34.15 (95% CI 27.13–70.53)	$p = 0.16$
In situ fixation	Yes (% of group)	2 (10.53%)	2 (16.67%)	$p = 0.63$
	No (% of group)	17 (89.47%)	10 (83.33%)	
Perioperative volume therapy (L)		1616 ± 661.2 (95% CI 1297–1934)	1291 ± 784.2 (95% CI 793.1–1790)	$p = 0.46$
Postoperative weight bearing	Partial weight bearing (% of group)	18 (94.74%)	10 (83.33%)	$p = 0.54$
	Full weight bearing (% of group)	1 (5.26%)	2 (16.67%)	
Discharge status	Stationary rehabilitation (% of group)	5 (26.32%)	7 (58.33%)	$p = 0.13$
	Home (% of group)	14 (73.68%)	5 (41.67%)	

Abbreviations: DHS, dynamic hip screw; FNS, femoral neck system; ASA, American Society of Anesthesiologists (physical status classification system); CCI, Charlson Comorbidity Index; TTS, time to surgery; CCD, centrum–collum–diaphyseal. * Fisher's exact test assessing fracture distribution differences between groups (Type I + II vs. Type III). ** Fisher's exact test assessing fracture distribution differences between groups (Type I + II vs. Type III + IV).

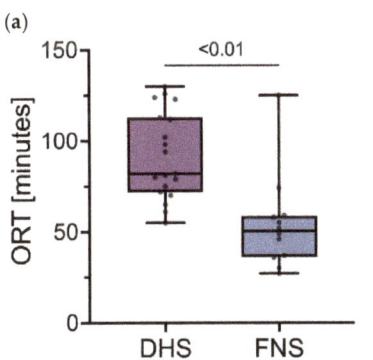
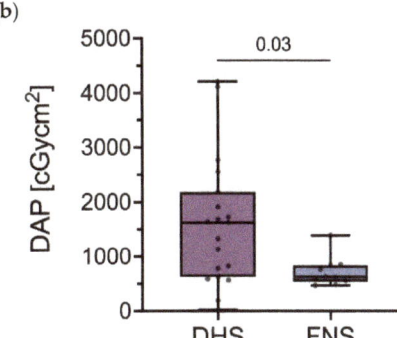

Figure 4. *Cont.*

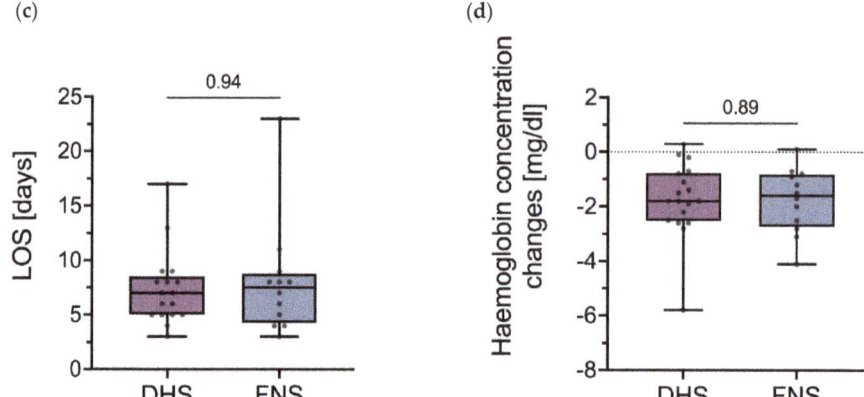

Figure 4. Outcome measures following osteosynthesis of FNF. (**a**) ORT, (**b**) DAP, (**c**) LOS, and (**d**) haemoglobin concentration changes in the DHS group and the FNS group. Abbreviations: FNF, femoral neck fracture; ORT, operating room time; DHS, dynamic hip screw; FNS, femoral neck system; DAP, dose-area product; LOS, length of stay.

4. Discussion

This study represents a comparative outcome analysis of two minimally invasive fixation systems used for the surgical management of FNF, namely the DHS with ARS and the FNS. This is the first study to employ broad inclusion criteria, as we assessed Garden type I to IV fractures and did not exclude any patients due to their pre-existing medical conditions. Compared to the DHS with ARS, perioperative outcome measures revealed a shorter ORT and lower DAP when using the FNS. There were no further differences between groups regarding the assessed outcomes. Particularly, there were no inter-group differences in the pre- and postoperative Pauwels and CCD angles between groups.

Fractures to the neck of the femur represent a relevant entity of the orthopaedic surgical spectrum [1]. Frequently, these injuries result in a life-changing event for patients, especially in geriatric cohorts [2]. Therefore, therapy concepts need to be highly efficient and straightforward to prevent adverse events [3] and to continuously improve the functional and patient-reported outcomes.

There is still an ongoing debate among orthopaedic specialists about whether patients may be eligible for reconstruction instead of an arthroplasty procedure. Various individual factors need to be considered, including the specific type of fracture and individual patient characteristics such as biological age, comorbidities, and previous mobility [4]. Furthermore, the typical complications of each of these approaches also need to be taken into account [21,22]. When considering DHS, infection rates of 1.3% have been reported [23].

Reconstruction is accepted in presumably intact femoral head perfusion and in biologically young patients. Non-displaced fractures in high-risk patients with multiple comorbidities also represent well-accepted indications for fixation. Since its introduction in 2018, the FNS has expanded the spectrum of available fixation systems [12–18,22,24]. It is assumed to be less invasive, thereby potentially reducing perioperative risks [10,11]. Published biomechanical data for the FNS demonstrate superiority compared to cannulated screws in Pauwels type III fractures [13]. Other studies have shown that the FNS might be more resistant to varus deformation, which is one of the main failure modes of femoral neck fixation [25].

However, there is still a lack of clinical outcome data for the FNS. Stassen et al. reported data with a maximum follow-up of one year after FNS implantation [24]. The authors included all FNF types. Multiple injured and patients with severe chronic medical conditions were excluded. The authors observed an ORT of 34 ± 9.4 min, incision sizes of

45.3 ± 8.8 mm, and an LOS of 4 ± 2.8 days. These data are in concordance with our results and corroborate the assumed less invasiveness of the FNS.

Other studies compared the FNS with three cannulated screws [14–16,18] and observed heterogeneous outcomes. He et al. reported shorter but not significantly different ORT, less radiation, a lower complication rate, and no differences in LOS [14]. Tang et al. confirmed the reduced fluoroscopy time in the FNS group [16]. However, the authors did not observe any significant differences in ORT, blood loss, incision size, or LOS. In contrast to these reports, Hu et al. and Zhou et al. reported longer ORT and higher blood loss when the FNS was used [15,18]. Furthermore, the LOS tended to be shorter, and patients had less pain and a shorter time to walk without crutches in the FNS group [18]. When discussing these data, one must consider that the latter two studies excluded typical patients: Hu et al. solely included patients under 60 years old and Zhou et al. excluded severely ill patients and patients with pre-existing severe cognitive dysfunction [15,18]. Hence, these studies may not reflect the typical, rising elderly patient cohort [4]. Partly, our results are in line with those of the aforementioned authors. We also observed reduced ORT and DAP, but our data do not allow for an adequate comparison of the previously reported blood loss reduction. At our clinic, the total amount of intraoperative blood loss was not systematically documented in the electronic medical data system. Therefore, we assessed differences in haemoglobin concentrations following surgery and perioperative volume management in order to take dilution into account. Here, we did not find any differences between groups. This may suggest that there was no significant difference in blood loss between groups, since haemoglobin differences and perioperatively administered fluids were not different and neither group needed a transfusion prior to hospital discharge. A reason for this could be that the total blood loss is dominated by the blood loss due to the initial trauma, making the additional blood loss due to the surgical procedure, either by DHS with ARS or by FNS, relatively minor.

To date, Vazquez et al. are the only authors that have compared the DHS, the FNS, and cannulated screws [17]. However, the authors only included Garden type I and II fractures in an elderly cohort (mean age, 84.9 years). While the ORT was significantly shorter in the FNS group, there were no statistically significant differences in the transfusion rate and LOS between groups. The absolute values of the ORT and LOS compare well to our results. Furthermore, we did not observe different transfusion rates since no patient needed transfusion.

In particular, the broadly observed decrease in the ORT is of utmost importance since published data show that prolonged ORT is associated with an increased risk of postoperative complications [26]. However, the most frequent surgical complication following the osteosynthesis of the FNF is the shortening of the femoral neck and the development of avascular necroses (AVN), which is observed in up to 20% of cases [27,28]. Accordingly, the data showed a conversion rate to arthroplasty in up to 10% of cases after osteosynthesis of the femoral neck [14,17,22]. Therefore, pre-existing comorbidities, such as osteoarthrosis of the hip, severe osteoporosis, rheumatoid arthritis, and chronic kidney disease, should be taken into account, as they confer a high risk of secondary osteosynthesis failure [29]. However, we did not observe any of these complications during the primary hospital stay, which was the focus of this report.

The current study has some limitations. First, the study groups were rather small, thereby potentially limiting the statistical power. This needs to be addressed in future studies through larger cohorts. However, published clinical data for the FNS are, thus far, rare, and we provide perioperative clinical data comparing the FNS with a commonly used implant in daily clinical practice. Furthermore, there were no broad exclusion criteria, either regarding fracture types or patient characteristics. Second, we were not able to contribute clinical outcome data exceeding the primary hospital stay. This limits the overall significance of our study. Therefore, further outcome data are needed to effectively assess long-term clinical outcomes and any subsequent complications. During the aforementioned study period, we did not observe any implant-associated complications. Nonetheless, future studies are needed to prospectively assess perioperative and long-term clinical, functional, and patient-reported outcomes to adequately compare osteosynthesis systems.

5. Conclusions

The FNS is a highly effective fixation system for the surgical management of FNF. It allows for a significant reduction in the duration of surgery, thereby potentially reducing surgery-related risks and complications.

Author Contributions: Conceptualisation, M.N. and F.G.; Methodology, M.N. and F.G.; Formal Analysis, M.N. and F.G., Investigation, M.N. and F.G.; Resources, K.F.B., S.S.A., U.S. and S.M.; Data Curation, M.N. and F.G.; Writing—Original Draft Preparation, M.N. and F.G.; Writing—Review & Editing, K.F.B., S.S.A., U.S. and S.M.; Visualisation, M.N.; Supervision, K.F.B. and F.G.; Project Administration, M.N. and F.G. All authors have read and agreed to the published version of the manuscript.

Funding: We acknowledge support from the German Research Foundation (DFG) and the Open Access Publication Fund of Charité—Universitätsmedizin Berlin (grant number 433849769).

Institutional Review Board Statement: The study was conducted according to the guidelines of the Declaration of Helsinki and approved by the local institutional ethics board (application number EA4/141/21, approved on the 17 June 2021).

Informed Consent Statement: Patient consent was waived due to the retrospective study character.

Data Availability Statement: The data presented in this study are available on request from the corresponding author. The data are not publicly available due to regulations of the local institutional ethics board.

Acknowledgments: We acknowledge the exceptional support of Erik Olm concerning the identification of eligible patients.

Conflicts of Interest: All authors report no conflict of interest.

References

1. Gullberg, B.; Johnell, O.; Kanis, J.A. World-wide projections for hip fracture. *Osteoporos Int.* **1997**, *7*, 407–413. Available online: https://pubmed.ncbi.nlm.nih.gov/9425497/ (accessed on 4 January 2022). [CrossRef] [PubMed]
2. Dyer, S.M.; Crotty, M.; Fairhall, N.; Magaziner, J.; Beaupre, L.A.; Cameron, I.D.; Sherrington, C. A critical review of the long-term disability outcomes following hip fracture. *BMC Geriatr.* **2016**, *16*, 158. Available online: https://pubmed.ncbi.nlm.nih.gov/27590604/ (accessed on 4 January 2022). [CrossRef] [PubMed]
3. Klestil, T.; Röder, C.; Stotter, C.; Winkler, B.; Nehrer, S.; Lutz, M.; Klerings, I.; Wagner, G.; Gartlehner, G.; Nussbaumer-Streit, B. Impact of timing of surgery in elderly hip fracture patients: A systematic review and meta-analysis. *Sci. Rep.* **2018**, *8*, 13933. Available online: https://pubmed.ncbi.nlm.nih.gov/30224765/ (accessed on 4 January 2022). [CrossRef] [PubMed]
4. Fischer, H.; Maleitzke, T.; Eder, C.; Ahmad, S.; Stöckle, U.; Braun, K.F. Management of proximal femur fractures in the elderly: Current concepts and treatment options. *Eur J Med Res.* **2021**, *26*, 86. Available online: https://pubmed.ncbi.nlm.nih.gov/34348796/ (accessed on 4 January 2022). [CrossRef] [PubMed]
5. Bhandari, M.; Swiontkowski, M. Management of Acute Hip Fracture. *N. Engl. J. Med.* **2017**, *377*, 2053–2062. Available online: https://pubmed.ncbi.nlm.nih.gov/29166235/ (accessed on 4 January 2022). [CrossRef]
6. Pauwels, F. Der Schenkelhalsbruch. In *Gesammelte Abhandlungen zur funktionellen Anat des Bewegungsapparates*; Springer: Berlin/Heidelberg, Germany, 1965; pp. 1–138. Available online: https://link.springer.com/chapter/10.1007/978-3-642-86841-2_1 (accessed on 2 February 2022).
7. Garden, R.S. Low-Angle Fixation in Fractures of the Femoral Neck. *J. Bone Jt. Surgery. Br. Vol.* **1961**, *43-B*, 647–663. Available online: https://online.boneandjoint.org.uk/doi/abs/10.1302/0301-620X.43B4.647 (accessed on 2 February 2022). [CrossRef]
8. Freitas, A.; Júnior, J.V.T.; dos Santos, A.F.; Aquino, R.J.; Leão, V.N.; de Alcântara, W.P. Biomechanical study of different internal fixations in Pauwels type III femoral neck fracture—A finite elements analysis. *J. Clin. Orthop. Trauma* **2021**, *14*, 145–150. [CrossRef]
9. Li, L.; Zhao, X.; Yang, X.; Tang, X.; Liu, M. Dynamic hip screws versus cannulated screws for femoral neck fractures: A systematic review and meta-analysis. *J. Orthop. Surg. Res.* **2020**, *15*, 352. Available online: https://pubmed.ncbi.nlm.nih.gov/32843048/ (accessed on 4 January 2022). [CrossRef]
10. DePuy Synthes. Femoral Neck System (FNS). 2019. Available online: https://www.jnjmedicaldevices.com/sites/default/files/user_uploaded_assets/pdf_assets/2019-09/FNSValueBrief.pdf (accessed on 4 January 2022).
11. DePuy Synthes. Femoral Neck System Operationstechnik. 2018. Available online: http://synthes.vo.llnwd.net/o16/LLNWMB8/INTMobile/SynthesInternational/ProductSupportMaterial/legacy_Synthes_PDF/DSEM-TRM-0614-0098-3a_LR.pdf (accessed on 4 January 2022).

12. Cha, Y.; Song, J.-U.; Yoo, J.-I.; Park, K.H.; Kim, J.-T.; Park, C.H.; Choy, W.-S. Improved control over implant anchorage under the use of the femoral neck system for fixation of femoral neck fractures: A technical note. *BMC Musculoskelet. Disord.* **2021**, *22*, 621. Available online: https://pubmed.ncbi.nlm.nih.gov/34256741/ (accessed on 4 January 2022). [CrossRef]
13. Stoffel, K.; Zderic, I.; Gras, F.; Sommer, C.; Eberli, U.; Mueller, M.; Oswald, M.; Gueorguiev, B. Biomechanical Evaluation of the Femoral Neck System in Unstable Pauwels III Femoral Neck Fractures: A Comparison with the Dynamic Hip Screw and Cannulated Screws. *J. Orthop. Trauma* **2017**, *31*, 131–137. Available online: https://pubmed.ncbi.nlm.nih.gov/27755333/ (accessed on 4 January 2022). [CrossRef] [PubMed]
14. He, C.; Lu, Y.; Wang, Q.; Ren, C.; Li, M.; Yang, M.; Xu, Y.; Li, Z.; Zhang, K.; Ma, T. Comparison of the clinical efficacy of a femoral neck system versus cannulated screws in the treatment of femoral neck fracture in young adults. *BMC Musculoskelet. Disord.* **2021**, *22*, 994. Available online: https://pubmed.ncbi.nlm.nih.gov/34844578/ (accessed on 4 January 2022). [CrossRef] [PubMed]
15. Hu, H.; Cheng, J.; Feng, M.; Gao, Z.; Wu, J.; Lu, S. Clinical outcome of femoral neck system versus cannulated compression screws for fixation of femoral neck fracture in younger patients. *J. Orthop. Surg. Res.* **2021**, *16*, 370. Available online: https://pubmed.ncbi.nlm.nih.gov/34107990/ (accessed on 4 January 2022). [CrossRef] [PubMed]
16. Tang, Y.; Zhang, Z.; Wang, L.; Xiong, W.; Fang, Q.; Wang, G. Femoral neck system versus inverted cannulated cancellous screw for the treatment of femoral neck fractures in adults: A preliminary comparative study. *J. Orthop. Surg. Res.* **2021**, *16*, 504. Available online: https://pubmed.ncbi.nlm.nih.gov/34399801/ (accessed on 4 January 2022). [CrossRef]
17. Vazquez, O.; Gamulin, A.; Hannouche, D.; Belaieff, W. Osteosynthesis of non-displaced femoral neck fractures in the elderly population using the femoral neck system (FNS): Short-term clinical and radiological outcomes. *J. Orthop. Surg. Res.* **2021**, *16*, 477. Available online: https://pubmed.ncbi.nlm.nih.gov/34348753/ (accessed on 4 January 2022). [CrossRef] [PubMed]
18. Zhou, X.-Q.; Li, Z.-Q.; Xu, R.-J.; She, Y.-S.; Zhang, X.-X.; Chen, G.-X.; Yu, X. Comparison of Early Clinical Results for Femoral Neck System and Cannulated Screws in the Treatment of Unstable Femoral Neck Fractures. *Orthop Surg.* **2021**, *13*, 1802–1809. Available online: https://pubmed.ncbi.nlm.nih.gov/34351048/ (accessed on 4 January 2022). [CrossRef] [PubMed]
19. Charlson, M.; Szatrowski, T.P.; Peterson, J.; Gold, J. Validation of a combined comorbidity index. *J. Clin. Epidemiol.* **1994**, *47*, 1245–1251. Available online: https://pubmed.ncbi.nlm.nih.gov/7722560/ (accessed on 4 January 2022). [CrossRef]
20. Motulsky, H.J.; Brown, R.E. Detecting outliers when fitting data with nonlinear regression—A new method based on robust nonlinear regression and the false discovery rate. *BMC Bioinform.* **2006**, *7*, 123. Available online: https://bmcbioinformatics.biomedcentral.com/articles/10.1186/1471-2105-7-123 (accessed on 3 February 2022). [CrossRef] [PubMed]
21. Chaplin, V.; Matharu, G.; Knebel, R. Complications following hemiarthroplasty for displaced intracapsular femoral neck fractures in the absence of routine follow-up. *Ann. R. Coll. Surg. Engl.* **2013**, *95*, 271–274. [CrossRef] [PubMed]
22. Cintean, R.; Pankratz, C.; Hofmann, M.; Gebhard, F.; Schütze, K. Early Results in Non-Displaced Femoral Neck Fractures Using the Femoral Neck System. *Geriatr. Orthop. Surg. Rehabil.* **2021**, *12*. Available online: https://pubmed.ncbi.nlm.nih.gov/34733579/ (accessed on 4 January 2022). [CrossRef] [PubMed]
23. HrubIna, M.; SkOták, M.; BěHOunek, J. Osteosyntéza zlomenin proximálního femuru metodou DHS: Infekční komplikace DHS Osteosynthesis for Proximal Femoral Fractures: Infectious Complications. *ACHOT* **2013**, *80*, 351–355.
24. Stassen, R.C.; Jeuken, R.M.; Boonen, B.; Meesters, B.; de Loos, E.R.; van Vugt, R. First clinical results of 1-year follow-up of the femoral neck system for internal fixation of femoral neck fractures. *Arch. Orthop. Trauma. Surg.* **2021**. Available online: https://pubmed.ncbi.nlm.nih.gov/34734328/ (accessed on 4 January 2022). [CrossRef]
25. Schopper, C.; Zderic, I.; Menze, J.; Müller, D.; Rocci, M.; Knobe, M.; Shoda, E.; Richards, G.; Gueorguiev, B.; Stoffel, K. Higher stability and more predictive fixation with the Femoral Neck System versus Hansson Pins in femoral neck fractures Pauwels II. *J. Orthop. Transl.* **2020**, *24*, 88–95. Available online: https://pubmed.ncbi.nlm.nih.gov/32775200/ (accessed on 4 January 2022). [CrossRef]
26. Cheng, H.; Clymer, J.W.; Chen, B.P.-H.; Sadeghirad, B.; Ferko, N.C.; Cameron, C.G.; Hinoul, P. Prolonged operative duration is associated with complications: A systematic review and meta-analysis. *J. Surg. Res.* **2018**, *229*, 134–144. [CrossRef] [PubMed]
27. Nanty, L.; Canovas, F.; Rodriguez, T.; Faure, P.; Dagneaux, L. Femoral neck shortening after internal fixation of Garden I fractures increases the risk of femoral head collapse. *Orthop. Traumatol. Surg. Res.* **2019**, *105*, 999–1004. [CrossRef] [PubMed]
28. Linde, F.; Andersen, E.; Hvass, I.; Madsen, F.; Pallesen, R. Avascular femoral head necrosis following fracture fixation. *Injury* **1986**, *17*, 159–163. [CrossRef]
29. Melisik, M.; Hrubina, M.; Daniel, M.; Cibula, Z.; Rovnak, M.; Necas, L. Ultra-short cementless anatomical stem for intracapsular femoral neck fractures in patients younger than 60 years. *Acta Orthop. Belg.* **2021**, *87*, 619–627. [CrossRef] [PubMed]

Article

Internal Fixation of Garden Type III Femoral Neck Fractures with Sliding Hip Screw and Anti-Rotation Screw: Does Increased Valgus Improve Healing?

Simon Hackl [1,2,*], Christian von Rüden [1,2], Ferdinand Weisemann [1], Isabella Klöpfer-Krämer [2,3], Fabian M. Stuby [1] and Florian Högel [1,2]

1 Department of Trauma Surgery, BG Unfallklinik Murnau, 82418 Murnau, Germany
2 Institute for Biomechanics, Paracelsus Medical University, 5020 Salzburg, Austria
3 Institute for Biomechanics, BG Unfallklinik Murnau, 82418 Murnau, Germany
* Correspondence: simon.hackl@bgu-murnau.de; Tel.: +49-8841-480

Abstract: *Background and Objectives:* The aim of this study was to compare the effect of valgus versus anatomic reduction on internal fixation of Garden type III femoral neck fractures using the sliding hip screw (SHS) and anti-rotation screw (ARS) regarding the radiographic and therapeutic outcome. *Patients and Methods:* A retrospective case-controlled study was performed in a level I trauma center. All patients between 2006 and 2020 aged younger than 70 years with a Garden type III femoral neck fracture and a Kellgren–Lawrence score under grade III stabilized using SHS and ARS were identified. One-hundred and nine patients were included, with a group distribution of sixty-eight patients in group A (anatomic reduction) and forty-one patients in group B (valgus reduction). *Results:* Mean age was 55 years, and the mean Kellgren–Lawrence score was 1 in both groups. Mean femoral neck angle was 130.5 ± 3.8° in group A and 142.8 ± 4.3° in group B ($p = 0.001$), with an over-correction of 12° in group B. Tip-apex distance was 10.0 ± 2.8 mm in group A versus 9.3 ± 2.8 mm in group B ($p = 0.89$). Healing time was 9 weeks in group A compared to 12 weeks in group B ($p = 0.001$). Failure rate was 4.4% in group A and 17.1% in group B ($p = 0.027$). *Conclusions:* Anatomic reduction of Garden type III femoral neck fractures in patients younger than 70 years treated using SHS and ARS resulted in significantly lower failure rates and shorter healing times than after valgus reduction. Therefore, it can be recommended to achieve anatomic reduction.

Keywords: femoral neck fracture; Garden classification; sliding hip screw; anti-rotation screw; valgus reduction; Kellgren–Lawrence score; outcome

1. Introduction

Younger adults are more likely to suffer from unstable Garden type III femoral neck fractures demanding accurate reduction and stable internal fixation, while having a higher likelihood of failure due to missing intrinsic instability [1–3]. Although there is still a lack of consensus regarding the most appropriate fixation technique for femoral neck fractures, sliding hip screw (SHS) supplemented with a cannulated anti-rotation screw (ARS) is commonly accepted as one of the gold standards for vertical fractures of the femoral neck in younger patients [4]. Apart from the anatomic reduction of these fracture configurations and the optimal restoration of the femoral neck-shaft angle (caput-collum-diaphyseal angle, CCD), the desirable or undesirable possibility of a valgus reduction occurs. In addition to total hip arthroplasty, in cases of failed fixation of femoral neck fractures, an often-described salvage procedure is valgus intertrochanteric osteotomy to achieve valgus positioning of the proximal fracture fragment [5]. Hereby, a larger CCD could be achieved, which converts shear forces at the femoral neck to compressive forces to improve osseous healing, resulting in suitable outcomes and adequate healing rates [5–8]. Consequently, a potential approach to further minimize complications and to maximize healing rates even in the initial surgical treatment of displaced femoral neck fractures might be to perform the fracture reduction in a slight valgus position of the proximal fragment prior to fracture fixation. Therefore, the aim of this study was to compare the effect of valgus alignment with the effect of anatomical reduction during closed internal fixation of Garden type III femoral neck fractures regarding the radiographic and therapeutic outcome, as well as the time period until osseous healing, using SHS combined with ARS. It was hypothesized that there would be faster and improved fracture healing and a better clinical outcome following valgus reduction of the fracture than after anatomic fracture reduction.

2. Patients and Methods

2.1. Study Design

A retrospective case-controlled study was performed in a single European level I trauma center. All patients between 2006 and 2020 aged younger than 70 years suffering a femoral neck fracture diagnosed by biplanar conventional radiographs and stabilized by using SHS combined with ARS were identified. Whenever conventional radiographs were not conclusive to determine the diagnosis or the classification of a femoral neck fracture, computed-tomography (CT) scan was performed to clarify the type of fracture. Garden classification was used to identify the fracture pattern [9]. To minimize inter-observer variation, all fractures were assessed by two experienced senior surgeons and only fractures that were identically classified by both surgeons were included [10]. To objectify the severity of the injury and the morbidity of the study group only patients with a Garden type III femoral neck fracture and a Kellgren-Lawrence score under grade III were included in the study after analyzing the radiological images taken on the day of accident [11–13]. Patients with preliminary disturbances of gait patterns and injuries of the affected hip as well as patients with an incomplete follow-up were excluded. After checking the mentioned inclusion and exclusion criteria, the data sets of 109 patients (age 55 ± 11 years; 63 males, 46 females) were included in the analysis (Figure 1).

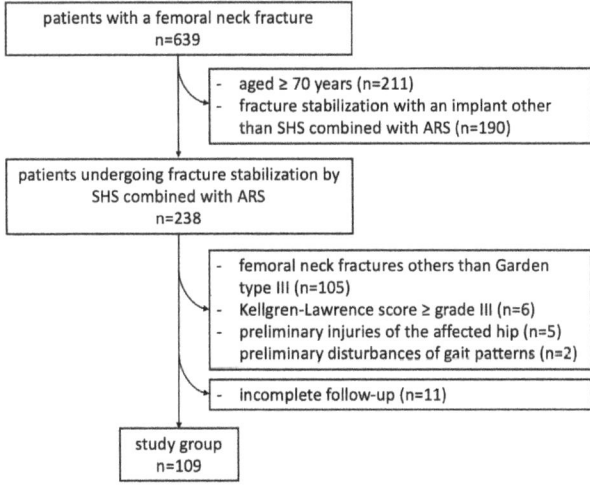

Figure 1. Overview on patients' inclusion process.

2.2. Surgical Procedure

All surgical procedures were performed in a standard manner under the supervision of twelve experienced senior surgeons. Patients were positioned on the extension table and closed reduction was performed either in anatomic or valgus position as decided by the surgeon—preoperatively and independently of individual patient and fracture criteria—with biplanar X-ray control. Following preparation to the proximal femur region and correct positioning of the aiming device for SHS, a 2.5 mm guide wire was placed center–center into the femoral head to the subchondral area. The position in the femoral neck was aimed to be in the caudal-dorsal quarter. After positioning of the guide wire and biplanar fluoroscopic control, a second 3.2 mm guide wire for the ARS was placed parallel to the first wire, cranially. After measuring the length of the SHS (DHS System, Synthes GmbH, Oberdorf, Switzerland), the femoral neck was prepared using the three-step drill, which was adjusted 10 mm shorter than the measured length following the insertion of the SHS over the guide wire. This procedure was followed by measuring the length of the ARS and insertion by using a cannulated 6.5 mm partial threaded screw (Asnis™ III, Stryker Trauma AG, Selzach, Switzerland), reaching the subchondral area, too. After removing the guide wires and after another X-ray control of the correct positioning of the SHS and ARS, the 2- or 4-hole SHS plate with a barrel angle of 130° or 135° (DHS System, Synthes GmbH, Oberdorf, Switzerland) was fixed to the SHS and the proximal femoral shaft with 2 or 4 bi-cortical 4.5 mm cortex screws. After surgical stabilization of the femoral neck, fracture pain-adapted full-weight-bearing was allowed for all patients.

2.3. Clinical and Radiological Assessment

As well as epidemiological patient parameters and the Kellgren–Lawrence score at the time of hospital admission, the femoral neck angles (°) were captured in comparison to the opposite side (Figure 2a) after reduction and surgical stabilization six weeks postoperatively by using biplanar conventional radiographs. Valgus reduction was defined as a femoral neck angle of more than 5° in comparison to the opposite side. Then, the cohort group was divided into group "A", which included patients with anatomical reduction, and group "B", which consisted of patients with valgus reduction of the Garden type III femoral neck fracture. Further on, the angle of the 2- or 4-hole SHS plate (°), the tip-apex distance (mm) as described by Baumgaertner et al. (Figure 2b), and the angle between SHS and ARS (°) were measured in frontal (Figure 2c) and axial planes (Figure 2d) of the intraoperative or postoperative X-rays [14].

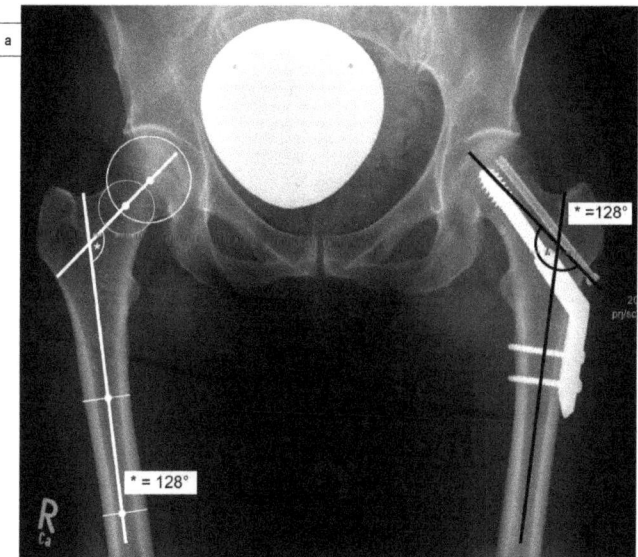

Figure 2. Cont.

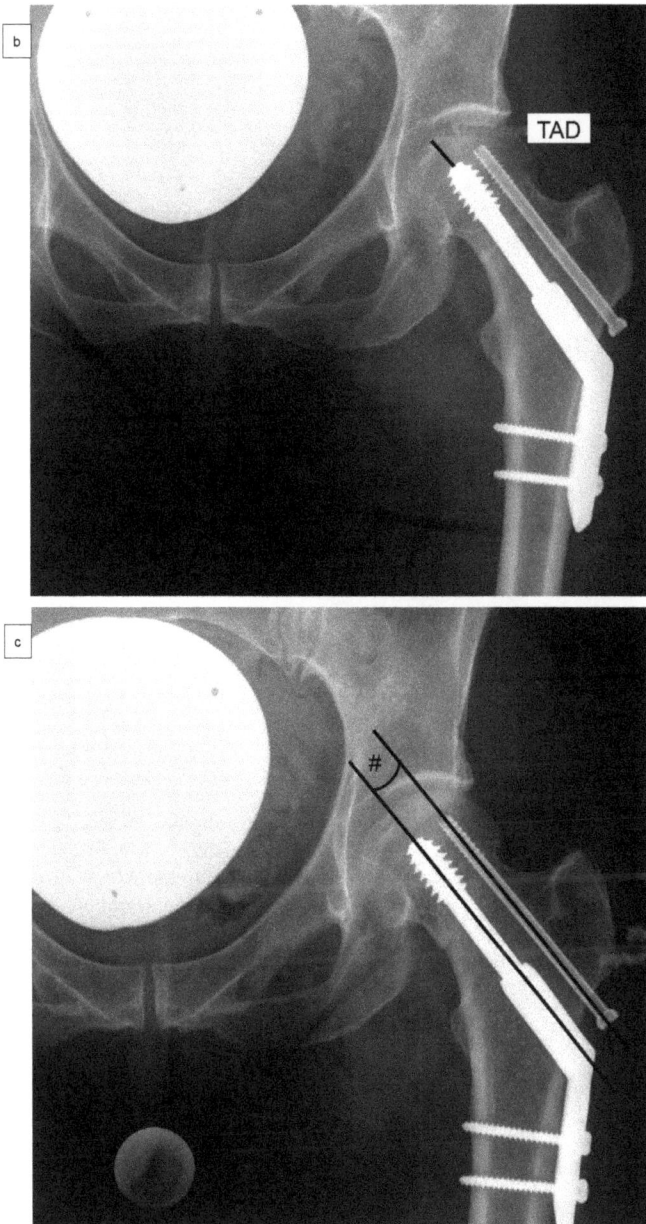

Figure 2. *Cont.*

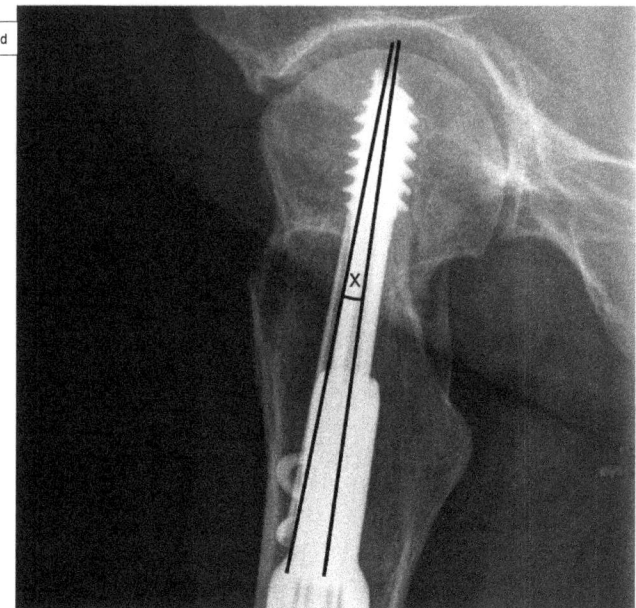

Figure 2. Measurement of the femoral neck angle (*) compared to the contralateral side (°), defined as the angle between the femoral neck axis and the bisecting line of the femoral shaft (**a**). The tip-apex distance (TAD) was defined as the calibrated summation of the distance between the tip of the SHS and the apex of the femoral head on anteroposterior and (not demonstrated) lateral radiographs (mm) (**b**), and the angle between SHS and ASR in the frontal plane (#) (**c**) and the axial plane (x) (**d**) by using biplanar conventional radiographs, six weeks postoperatively.

In each follow-up visit, the healing time (weeks) and failure rate as well as potential surgery-related complications were examined. Hereby, treatment failure was defined as cutting out of the SHS, and respectively the ARS, collapse of the femoral head, implant loosening, or failure of fracture healing up to 6 months after surgical stabilization. Fracture healing was defined as osseous union of at least three cortices diagnosed by biplanar conventional radiographs [15].

2.4. Follow-Up

After discharge from the hospital, patients were followed-up clinically and radiologically in the outpatient department at regular intervals after 6 weeks, followed by 4-week intervals until the sixth month after surgical stabilization of the femoral neck fracture or until fracture healing was documented. In addition, in case of suspected complications, additional visits were scheduled. During each visit, patients where clinically and radiologically examined regarding fracture healing and possible complications. Furthermore, in addition to these documented follow-up examinations, the conventional radiographs were retrospectively re-evaluated by two experienced senior surgeons to verify the healing time, defined as the time from the diagnosis of the femoral neck fracture to its osseous consolidation.

2.5. Statistical Analysis

As well as implant-related parameters, tip-apex distance, Kellgren–Lawrence score, healing time and treatment failure were compared between groups A and B (SPSS version 26.0, SPSS Inc., Chicago, IL, USA). For all variables, a check for normal distribution was performed using the Kolmogorov–Smirnov test. Only two variables from the group of valgus patients (group B) demonstrated a normal distribution, so the non-parametric Mann–

Whitney test was used. Due to multiple testing, for the comparison of the three variables healing time, femoral neck angle and tip-apex distance, the significance level was set to $\alpha = 0.05/3 = 0.017$. The complications (dichotomous yes/no) were tested for a significant difference between the groups using Pearson's chi-square test ($\alpha = 0.05$). Effect sizes for significant differences were calculated using Cohen's d (for the Mann–Whitney test) and Phi's r (for Pearson's chi-square test) [16]. Results of this study are presented as mean values ± standard deviation. Results were considered statistically significant with p values < 0.05.

2.6. Ethics and Study Registration

The study adhered to the tenets of the Helsinki Declaration and according to the guidelines and the approval of the Ethics Committee of the institutional and national Medical Board (Bavarian State Chamber of Physicians, ID 2022-1157). On 2 August 2022, the study was retrospectively registered with the German Clinical Trials Register (Trial registration number: DRKS00029953).

3. Results

3.1. Patient Cohort

One-hundred and nine patients were included in the study, with a group distribution of sixty-eight patients in group A with anatomical and forty-one patients in group B with valgus reduction of the Garden type III femoral neck fracture (Table 1).

Table 1. Overview of the patient cohort with Garden type III femoral neck fractures divided into group A (anatomic reduction) and group B (valgus reduction). Values are presented as mean ± standard deviation or as total number of patients.

	Group A	Group B	*p*-Value
Group size	68	41	
Male	40	23	
Female	28	18	
Age	55 ± 11 years	55 ± 11 years	0.78
Body mass index	24.9 ± 3.2 kg/m^2	23.6 ± 3.5 kg/m^2	0.07
ASA [1]	1.6 ± 0.7	1.8 ± 0.6	0.26
Duration between trauma and fracture stabilization			
≤24 h	65	40	
>24 h	3	1	
SHS plate			
2-hole	61	38	
4-hole	7	3	
Barrel angle of SHS			
130°	7	3	
135°	61	38	
Kellgren–Lawrence score	1.0 ± 0.6	1.2 ± 0.6	0.14
Cut-to-seam time of the surgical procedure	58 ± 19 min	60 ± 21 min	0.70
Tip-apex distance (TAD)	10.0 ± 2.9 mm	9.3 ± 2.8 mm	0.89
Angle between SHS and ARS in frontal plane	0.0 ± 0.2°	0.0 ± 0.3°	0.56
Angle between SHS and ARS in axial plane	2.2 ± 1.8°	2.4 ± 1.5°	0.76
Femoral neck angle 6 weeks postoperatively	130.5 ± 3.8°	142.8 ± 4.3°	0.001
Difference of the femoral neck angle 6 weeks postoperatively in comparison to the contralateral side	1.2 ± 1.3°	12.0 ± 4.2°	0.001

[1] American Society of Anesthesiologists physical status classification.

The average femoral neck angle was significantly different between groups A and B (group A: 130.5 ± 3.8°, group B: 142.8 ± 4.3°; $p = 0.001$, effect size d = 0.829). In accordance with the inclusion criteria, the over-correction in comparison to the opposite side was performed with 12 ± 4.2° in group B and 1.2 ± 1.3° in group A ($p = 0.001$). Average age was 55 years in both groups (group A: 55 ± 11 years, group B: 55 ± 11 years). In addition, with an average Kellgren–Lawrence score of 1 in both groups, no significant difference could be observed (group A: 1.0 ± 0.6, group B: 1.2 ± 0.6). Regarding the tip-apex distance with 10.0 ± 2.9 mm in group A versus 9.3 ± 2.8 mm in group B ($p = 0.89$), no significant difference could be detected. In the axial plane of the biplanar X-rays, the mean angle between SHS and ARS in group A was 2.2 ± 1.8°, and 2.4 ± 1.5° in group B ($p = 0.76$). In the frontal plane of the biplanar X-rays, the screws were almost exactly parallel in both groups (group A: 0.0 ± 0.2°, group B: 0.0 ± 0.3°; $p = 0.56$). Considering the duration of the surgical procedure—defined by cut-to-seam time—as a parameter for its difficulty, no significant difference could be observed in both groups (group A: 58 ± 19 min, group B: 60 ± 21 min; $p = 0.70$).

3.2. Treatment Failure

Regarding the failure rate of the surgical-stabilized femoral neck fractures, a relevant difference could be observed between patients who received an anatomical and those who received a valgus reposition. The failure rate was significantly higher in group B than in group A, as 7 complications (17.1%) appeared after valgus reduction in group B and 3 cases with fracture-related complications (4.4%) were detected after anatomical reduction in group A ($p = 0.027$, effect size r = 0.212) (Figure 3).

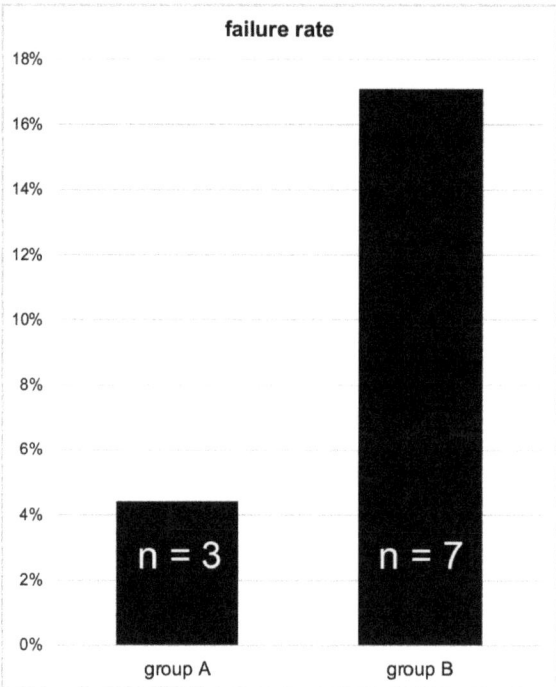

Figure 3. Comparison of the failure rate in surgically treated Garden type III femoral neck fractures.

In detail, in group A, two cases of femoral head necrosis were observed, while one of these cases was stabilized more than 24 h after trauma and one cutting out of the SHS was found. In group B, femoral head necrosis was found in five cases and cutting out of the

SHS in two cases. All these patients had to be revised by total hip arthroplasty (THA) due to immobilizing hip pain. Implant loosening or failure of the fracture to heal over 6 months were not observed in any patient.

3.3. Healing Time

In accordance with the above-mentioned treatment failure, osseous healing of the Garden type III femoral neck fracture stabilized by SHS and ARS could be achieved in group A in 65 out of 68 patients and in group B in 34 out of 41 patients during the follow-up period of 6 months, accompanied by full-weight-bearing. Hereby, osseous healing was significantly shorter after anatomical reduction in group A, with a mean healing time of 9 ± 2 weeks compared to 12 ± 2 weeks after valgus reposition in group B ($p = 0.001$, effect size d = 0.509) (Figure 4).

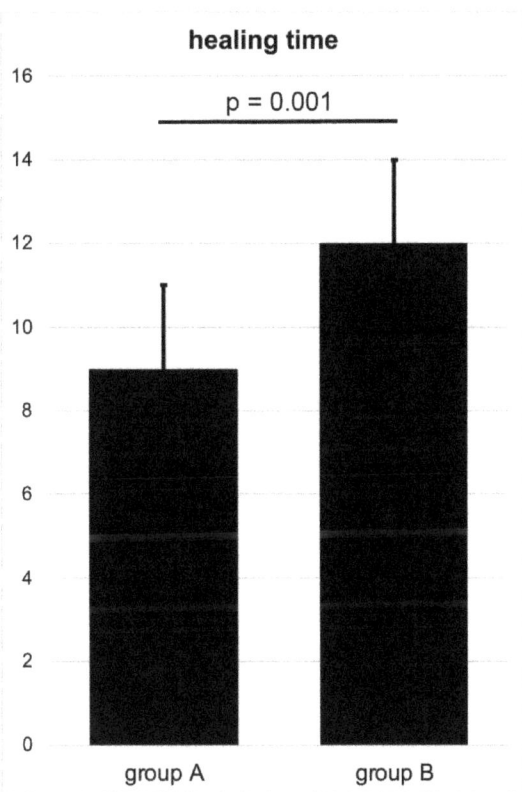

Figure 4. Duration of time to osseous healing after anatomical and valgus reduction stabilized using SHS and ARS (weeks) in a Garden type III femoral neck fracture.

4. Discussion

The objective of this study was to evaluate the potential influence of valgus reduction on the healing process in Garden type III femoral neck fractures fixed using SHS in combination with ARS. Despite the promising outcome of valgus intertrochanteric osteotomy as well as biomechanical considerations, performing the fracture reduction in Garden type III femoral neck fractures in a slight valgus position of the proximal fragment prior to fracture fixation with SHS and ARS was not superior compared with the anatomical reduction in patients younger than 70 years. In the current study, an average valgus correction of femoral neck fractures of 12° resulted in a significantly increased rate of treatment failure as well as in a longer period of time until fracture healing of about 3 months. In so far, based on the results of this study in patients younger than 70 years, anatomical reduction of Garden type III femoral neck fractures is suggested prior to internal fixation with SHS and ARS.

There are several studies examining the outcome and the biomechanical behavior after femoral neck fractures regarding the different types of fracture fixation, demonstrating an advantage of the sliding hip screw systems in combination with an additional anti-rotation screw [1,17]. Nevertheless, studies regarding the influence of the reduction of the proximal fragment of femoral neck fractures are rare and difficult to compare due to the different methods of fracture stabilization. Regardless of this, femoral neck fractures fixed in a varus position demonstrated the highest rate of failure (37.5%), followed by fractures fixed with a visible medial transcervical line independent of anatomical or valgus reduction of the proximal fragment (36.0%) [18]. In a recently published finite element analysis, anatomic reduction of valgus-impacted femoral neck fractures diminished the stress at the fracture ends, although displacement significantly increased. When the fracture was fixed with SHS and ARS, there was less stress at the fracture end with anatomic reduction than without [19]. For example, Ramallo et al. examined 81 patients younger than 60 years with femoral neck fractures treated with closed reduction and internal fixation using three cannulated screws and evaluated a significant influence of a satisfactory reduction on the outcome [20]. Satisfactory reduction was defined as deviation of the focus of the fracture less than 2 mm in combination with Garden angles between 160° and 180°. After sufficient reduction, treatment failure was observed in 7% compared with an over 8 times higher risk of failure when the reduction was inadequate. Although the failure rate of satisfactory reductions was comparable to our failure rate of 4% after anatomic reduction, no statement was made regarding valgus positioning by Ramallo et al. [20]. Schwartsmann et al. detected a failure rate in femoral neck fractures after good reduction—defined by a normal or slightly valgus reduction in accordance with the alignment index stated by Garden—and stabilization with a sliding hip screw system in about 20% of the cases, comparable to our failure rate of 17.5% after valgus reduction [21,22]. Incorrect screw positioning in the femoral head was identified as a main risk factor for therapy failure due to necrosis [21]. A comparable failure rate of 19.5% to the valgus group of the current study was observed after fixation of femoral neck fractures with valgus impaction and any further reduction [23]. Although there are studies which did not find any affection of the healing rate by the quality of reduction [24,25], failure rates in the present study correlate with the majority of the current literature, highlighting the need of an appropriate reduction of femoral neck fractures. A closer look at the type of complications showed that in total, 7 out of 109 patients analyzed (6.4%) developed femoral head necrosis. In particular, after anatomic reduction, femoral head necrosis occurred in only 2 of 68 patients (2.9%) and after valgus reduction in 5 of 41 patients (12.2%) during follow-up. Considering the frequency of avascular necrosis of the femoral head after stabilization of Garden type III femoral neck fractures in the current literature, with a 95% confidence interval between 6.4% and 27.6%, the incidence of femoral head necrosis in our study cohort is quite low, especially after anatomic reduction [26]. One possible reason for this moderate necrosis rate could be—as noted in a recent meta-analysis—that femoral neck systems present a lower rate of femoral head necrosis than cannulated cancellous screws, which are also commonly used worldwide and thus may have an impact on the previously observed necrosis rates [27].

A more detailed look at the group of patients with an acceptable reduction of the femoral neck fracture demonstrated a mixed picture in the available literature: A study published in 1981 after evaluation of 446 cases of femoral neck fractures in all Garden's stages treated by internal fixation reported a healing rate of 90% after a reduction in valgus position and only 77% if anatomical reduction was achieved [28]. In addition, Füchtmeier et al. analyzed a patient cohort of 51 patients during 1975 and 1985 and reported that the anatomical reduction of femoral neck fractures—compared to a valgus position—and stabilization with mainly three to four cannulated screws resulted in a higher, but statistically not significant, rate of osteonecrosis (18.2%) and nonunion (9.1%) in the first 5 years following osteosynthesis [29]. These findings are in contrast to the present study, demonstrating a lower rate of treatment failure after anatomical reduction, with 4%, which is more interesting since in both studies, the average valgus correction of femoral neck fractures was about 12°. One possible explanation for these opposite findings might be the utilized stabilization with SHS and ARS instead of mainly cannulated screws, as well as that the patients' cohort includes all Garden's stages with a significantly higher rate of Garden type III femoral neck fractures in the group with valgus position. Looking at the group of patients with anatomical reduction between 5 and 15 years after internal fixation analyzed by Füchtmeier et al., a change in both groups was observed, and a better long-term outcome with an improved functional outcome and a lower rate of osteoarthritis of the hip were detected in the group that received anatomic reduction [29]. Focusing on therapy failure by analyzing 202 patients with femoral neck fractures treated using 3 cannulated screws, Yang et al. did not find any significant difference regarding development of nonunion after anatomical reduction [30]. Looking at the failure rate in relation to the size of the valgus tilt of valgus-impacted femoral neck fractures which were not dis-impacted and were stabilized with three cannulated screws, Song et al. could demonstrate that a valgus tilt above 15° results in a higher failure rate [31].

Another important point that supports the anatomical reduction of femoral neck fractures in addition to the above-mentioned lower risk of developing osteoarthritis of the hip in younger patients is the higher rate of femoral neck shortening in valgus-impacted femoral neck fracture combined with a worse functional outcome due to a femoral offset shortening and the resulting change in the abductor moment arm [31]. This is also emphasized by a study conducted by Park et al., which demonstrated that anatomical reduction of femoral neck fractures with valgus impaction above 15° leads to a better functional outcome one and two years following osteosynthesis, compared to in situ stabilization of the valgus-impacted femoral neck fractures without any reduction [25].

Relevant literature data regarding the time period between surgery and fracture healing could not be found yet. The results of the present study demonstrated a significantly shorter healing time after anatomic reduction of the femoral neck, which may be explained by less compromise of blood supply than after valgus reduction of the femoral neck.

Limitations of this study might be seen in the retrospective study design, resulting in a lack of clarity as to why in every single case, the surgical team decided for anatomical or valgus reduction. Besides, a longer follow-up for at least one year would be helpful to investigate if early secondary THA would have been needed due to the offset change related to the femoral neck angle reduction. Nevertheless, to our knowledge, the current study is the first clinical trial comparing SHS in combination with additive ARS in an excellent comparable patients' cohort consisting only of Garden type III femoral neck fracture stabilized by the same implants, with a focus on the intraoperative reduction angle of the femoral neck.

5. Conclusions

Anatomic reduction of Garden type III femoral neck fractures in patients younger than 70 years treated using SHS in combination with ARS resulted in significantly lower failure rates and shorter healing times than after valgus reduction between 5° and 15° of the proximal fracture fragment. Therefore, based on the results of the current study, it can be recommended to aim for anatomic reduction when using SHS and ARS for internal stabilization.

Author Contributions: Conceptualization, F.H.; Formal analysis, F.W. and I.K.-K.; Investigation, S.H. and F.H.; Methodology, F.H.; Validation, S.H. and F.H.; Visualization, S.H.; Writing—original draft, S.H., C.v.R. and F.H.; Writing—review & editing, S.H., C.v.R., F.W., I.K.-K., F.M.S. and F.H. All authors have read and agreed to the published version of the manuscript.

Funding: This research received no external funding.

Institutional Review Board Statement: The study was conducted in accordance with the Declaration of Helsinki and approved by the Ethics Committee of the institutional and national Medical Board (Bavarian State Chamber of Physicians, ID 2022-1157). On 2 August 2022, the study was retrospectively registered with the German Clinical Trials Register (Trial registration number: DRKS00029953).

Informed Consent Statement: Informed consent was obtained from all subjects involved in the study.

Data Availability Statement: The data presented in this study are available on request from the corresponding author. The data are not publicly available due to privacy.

Conflicts of Interest: The authors declare no conflict of interest.

References

1. Augat, P.; Bliven, E.; Hackl, S. Biomechanics of Femoral Neck Fractures and Implications for Fixation. *J. Orthop. Trauma* **2019**, *33* (Suppl. 1), S27–S32. [CrossRef] [PubMed]
2. Liporace, F.; Gaines, R.; Collinge, C.; Haidukewych, G.J. Results of internal fixation of Pauwels type-3 vertical femoral neck fractures. *J. Bone Jt. Surg.* **2008**, *90*, 1654–1659. [CrossRef] [PubMed]
3. Ly, T.V.; Swiontkowski, M.F. Treatment of femoral neck fractures in young adults. *J. Bone Jt. Surg.* **2008**, *90*, 2254–2266.
4. Bliven, E.; Sandriesser, S.; Augat, P.; von Rüden, C.; Hackl, S. Biomechanical evaluation of locked plating fixation for unstable femoral neck fractures. *Bone Jt. Res.* **2020**, *9*, 314–321. [CrossRef] [PubMed]
5. Yuan, B.J.; Shearer, D.W.; Barei, D.P.; Nork, S.E. Intertrochanteric Osteotomy for Femoral Neck Nonunion: Does "Undercorrection" Result in an Acceptable Rate of Femoral Neck Union? *J. Orthop. Trauma* **2017**, *31*, 420–426. [CrossRef] [PubMed]
6. Augat, P.; Hollensteiner, M.; von Rüden, C. The role of mechanical stimulation in the enhancement of bone healing. *Injury* **2021**, *52* (Suppl. 2), S78–S83. [CrossRef]
7. Min, B.-W.; Bae, K.-C.; Kang, C.-H.; Song, K.S.; Kim, S.-Y.; Won, Y.-Y. Valgus intertrochanteric osteotomy for non-union of femoral neck fracture. *Injury* **2006**, *37*, 786–790. [CrossRef]
8. Prakash, J.; Keshari, V.; Chopra, R.K. Experience of valgus osteotomy for neglected and failed osteosynthesis in fractures neck of femur. *Int. Orthop.* **2020**, *44*, 705–713. [CrossRef]
9. Kazley, J.M.; Banerjee, S.; Abousayed, M.M.; Rosenbaum, A.J. Classifications in Brief: Garden Classification of Femoral Neck Fractures. *Clin. Orthop. Relat. Res.* **2018**, *476*, 441–445. [CrossRef]
10. Frandsen, P.; Andersen, E.; Madsen, F.; Skjødt, T. Garden's classification of femoral neck fractures. An assessment of inter-observer variation. *J. Bone Jt. Surgery. Br.* **1988**, *70*, 588–590. [CrossRef]
11. Sjöholm, P.; Sundkvist, J.; Wolf, O.; Sköldenberg, O.; Gordon, M.; Mukka, S. Preoperative Anterior and Posterior Tilt of Garden I-II Femoral Neck Fractures Predict Treatment Failure and Need for Reoperation in Patients Over 60 Years. *JBJS Open Access* **2021**, *6*, e21.00045. [CrossRef] [PubMed]
12. Nyholm, A.M.; Palm, H.; Sandholdt, H.; Troelsen, A.; Gromov, K.; DFDB Collaborators. Risk of reoperation within 12 months following osteosynthesis of a displaced femoral neck fracture is linked mainly to initial fracture displacement while risk of death may be linked to bone quality: A cohort study from Danish Fracture Database. *Acta Orthop.* **2019**, *91*, 1–75. [CrossRef] [PubMed]
13. Kohn, M.D.; Sassoon, A.A.; Fernando, N.D. Classifications in Brief: Kellgren-Lawrence Classification of Osteoarthritis. *Clin. Orthop. Relat. Res.* **2016**, *474*, 1886–1893. [CrossRef] [PubMed]
14. Baumgaertner, M.R.; Curtin, S.L.; Lindskog, D.M.; Keggi, J.M. The value of the tip-apex distance in predicting failure of fixation of peritrochanteric fractures of the hip. *J. Bone Jt. Surg.* **1995**, *77*, 1058–1064. [CrossRef]
15. Fisher, J.S.; Kazam, J.J.; Fufa, D.; Bartolotta, R.J. Radiologic evaluation of fracture healing. *Skelet. Radiol.* **2019**, *48*, 349–361. [CrossRef]
16. Cohen, J. *Statistical Power Analysis for the Behavioral Sciences*, 2nd ed.; L. Lawrence Earlbaum Associates: Hillsdale, NJ, USA, 1988.
17. Samsami, S.; Augat, P.; Rouhi, G. Stability of femoral neck fracture fixation: A finite element analysis. *Proc. Inst. Mech. Eng. Part H* **2019**, *233*, 892–900. [CrossRef]
18. Kane, C.; Jo, J.; Siegel, J.; Matuszewski, P.E.; Swart, E. Can we predict failure of percutaneous fixation of femoral neck fractures? *Injury* **2020**, *51*, 357–360. [CrossRef]
19. Dai, Y.; Ni, M.; Dou, B.; Wang, Z.; Zhang, Y.; Cui, X.; Ma, W.; Qin, T.; Xu, X.; Mei, J. Finite element analysis of necessity of reduction and selection of internal fixation for valgus-impacted femoral neck fracture. *Comput. Methods Biomech. Biomed. Eng.* **2022**, 1–8. [CrossRef]
20. Ramallo, D.A.; Kropf, L.L.; Zaluski, A.D.; Cavalcanti, A.D.S.; Duarte, M.E.L.; Guimarães, J.A.M. Factors Influencing the Outcome of Osteosynthesis in the Fracture of the Femoral Neck in Young Adult Patients. *Rev. Bras. Ortop.* **2019**, *54*, 408–415. [CrossRef]
21. Schwartsmann, C.R.; Jacobus, L.S.; Spinelli, L.D.F.; Boschin, L.C.; Gonçalves, R.Z.; Yépez, A.K.; Barreto, R.P.G.; Silva, M.F. Dynamic hip screw for the treatment of femoral neck fractures: A prospective study with 96 patients. *ISRN Orthop.* **2014**, *2014*, 257871. [CrossRef]
22. Garden, R.S. Malreduction and avascular necrosis in subcapital fractures of the femur. *J. Bone Jt. Surgery. Br.* **1971**, *53*, 183–197. [CrossRef]

23. Moon, N.H.; Shin, W.C.; Jang, J.H.; Seo, H.U.; Bae, J.Y.; Suh, K.T. Surgical Outcomes of Internal Fixation Using Multiple Screws in Femoral Neck Fractures with Valgus Impaction: When Should We Consider Hip Arthroplasty? A Retrospective, Multicenter Study. *Hip Pelvis* **2019**, *31*, 136–143. [CrossRef]
24. Lindequist, S.; Törnkvist, H. Quality of reduction and cortical screw support in femoral neck fractures. An analysis of 72 fractures with a new computerized measuring method. *J. Orthop. Trauma* **1995**, *9*, 215–221. [CrossRef] [PubMed]
25. Park, Y.-C.; Um, K.-S.; Kim, D.-J.; Byun, J.; Yang, K.-H. Comparison of femoral neck shortening and outcomes between in situ fixation and fixation after reduction for severe valgus-impacted femoral neck fractures. *Injury* **2021**, *52*, 569–574. [CrossRef]
26. Konarski, W.; Poboży, T.; Kotela, A.; Śliwczyński, A.; Kotela, I.; Hordowicz, M.; Krakowiak, J. The Risk of Avascular Necrosis Following the Stabilization of Femoral Neck Fractures: A Systematic Review and Meta-Analysis. *Int. J. Environ. Res. Public Health* **2022**, *19*, 10050. [CrossRef] [PubMed]
27. Tian, P.; Kuang, L.; Li, Z.-J.; Xu, G.-J.; Fu, X. Comparison Between Femoral Neck Systems and Cannulated Cancellous Screws in Treating Femoral Neck Fractures: A Meta-Analysis. *Geriatr. Orthop. Surg. Rehabil.* **2022**, *13*, 21514593221113533. [CrossRef] [PubMed]
28. Nieminen, S.; Nurmi, M.; Satokari, K. Healing of femoral neck fractures; influence of fracture reduction and age. *Ann. Chir. Gynaecol.* **1981**, *70*, 26–31.
29. Hente, R.; Maghsudi, M.; Nerlich, M. Reposition der Schenkelhalsfraktur des jüngeren Menschen. Valgus- oder anatomische Reposition? [Repositioning femoral neck fracture in younger patients. Valgus or anatomic reposition?]. *Der Unfallchirurg* **2001**, *104*, 1055–1060. (In German) [CrossRef]
30. Yang, J.-J.; Lin, L.-C.; Chao, K.-H.; Chuang, S.-Y.; Wu, C.-C.; Yeh, T.-T.; Lian, Y.-T. Risk factors for nonunion in patients with intracapsular femoral neck fractures treated with three cannulated screws placed in either a triangle or an inverted triangle configuration. *J. Bone Jt. Surg. Am.* **2013**, *95*, 61–69. [CrossRef]
31. Song, H.K.; Lee, J.J.; Oh, H.C.; Yang, K.H. Clinical implication of subgrouping in valgus femoral neck fractures: Comparison of 31-B1.1 with 31-B1.2 fractures using the OTA/AO classification. *J. Orthop. Trauma* **2013**, *27*, 677–682. [CrossRef]

Article

High Percentage of Complications and Re-Operations Following Dynamic Locking Plate Fixation with the Targon® FN for Intracapsular Proximal Femoral Fractures: An Analysis of Risk Factors

Emanuel Kuner [1], Jens Gütler [2], Dimitri E. Delagrammaticas [3], Bryan J. M. van de Wall [1], Matthias Knobe [1], Frank J. P. Beeres [1,*], Reto Babst [1] and Björn-Christian Link [1]

1. Department of Orthopedic and Trauma Surgery, Lucerne Cantonal Hospital, 6000 Lucerne, Switzerland
2. Department of Orthopedics and Traumatology, Zug Cantonal Hospital, 6340 Baar, Switzerland
3. Central Coast Orthopedic Medical Group, 862 Meinecke Avenue, Suite 100, San Luis Obispo, CA 93405, USA
* Correspondence: frank.beeres@luks.ch; Tel.: +41-41-2051914

Abstract: The ideal surgical treatment of femoral neck fractures remains controversial. When treating these fractures with internal fixation, many fixation constructs exist. The primary aim of this study was to evaluate the incidence and specific risk factors associated with complication and re-operation following fixation of intracapsular proximal femoral fractures using the Targon-FN system (B.Braun Melsungen AG). A secondary aim was to identify if lateral prominence of the implant relative to the lateral border of the vastus ridge was a specific risk factor for elective plate removal. Methodically, a retrospective case series was conducted of all consecutive adult patients treated at a single level 1 trauma center in Switzerland for an intracapsular proximal femoral fracture with the Targon-FN. Demographic data were collected. Patients with a follow-up of less than three months were excluded. Complications as well as plate position were recorded. Statistical analysis to identify specific risk factors for re-operation and complications was performed. In result, a total of 72 cases with intracapsular femoral neck fractures were treated with the Targon-FN locking plate system between 2010 and 2017. Thirty-four patients (47.2%) experienced one or more complications. The most common complication was mechanical irritation of the iliotibial band (ITB) (23.6%, $n = 17$). Complications included intraarticular screw perforation (6.9%, n = 5), avascular necrosis (5.6%, n = 4), non-union (5.6%, n = 4) among others. In total, 46 re-operations were required. Younger age, fracture displacement and time to postoperative weight bearing were identified as risk factors for re-operation. In conclusion, intracapsular femoral neck fractures treated with the Targon-FN system resulted in a high rate of post-operative complication and re-operation. Statistical analysis revealed patient age, fracture displacement, time to postoperative full weight bearing were risk factors for re-operation. The main limitation is the limited number of cases and a short follow-up of less than 12 months in a subgroup of our patients.

Keywords: avascular; band; femoral; fracture; neck; necrosis; iliotibial; implant; osteosynthesis

1. Introduction

Femoral neck fractures are among the most common orthopaedic injuries treated in the elderly population [1]. In patients over 65 years of age, the incidence of femoral neck fractures is estimated to be between 600 and 900 per per year [2].

While arthroplasty is the preferred treatment in elderly patients with displaced intracapsular proximal femur fractures, in younger patients or stable fracture patterns in the elderly, joint preserving treatment with internal fixation may be favored [3–8]. However, complications that can occur after internal fixation, including excessive fracture shortening, varus collapse, avascular necrosis, and screw perforation leave room for improvement with internal fixation treatment methods [9–14]. Furthermore, variability among observed failures of the implants utilized for internal fixation of intracapsular hip fractures suggests an opportunity for optimization of implant design [9–11,15,16]. Both, cannulated femoral neck screws as well as the concept of sliding hip screws find many supporters. Biomechanically, the sliding hip screw concept appears to be more stable [17]. On the other hand, blood flow in the femoral head may be less impaired by cannulated femoral neck screws [18]. The large-scale FAITH trial was unable to give a qualified recommendation for one of the surgical techniques over the other [19]. In this context, the question arises whether a combination of concepts such as the Targon® FN (B.Braun AG, Melsungen, Germany) could constitute a superior construct resulting in improved outcome.

In 2007, the Targon® FN system (B.Braun AG, 34209 Melsungen, Germany) was developed by Parker MJ et al., which integrated a telescoping mechanism in each of the head-neck screws (TeleScrew), aimed at allowing more controlled fracture collapse and minimizing the risk of cut-through or backing out of screws. Moreover, locking fixation to the femoral shaft provides greater rotational stability to the construct. Rotational instability and strength of femoral head fixation have shown to be associated with tendencies for femoral neck shortening, fracture collapse, and construct failure [12].

Several studies have shown promising early results regarding complications, nonunion, and revision rates when using the Targon FN System [20–23]. In particular, the Targon FN system has shown promise in terms of lower risk of revision or re-operation compared to traditional cannulated screw fixation methods [21,24–26]. Other studies, however, report equivocal rates of complications with this implant compared to the established treatment standards including cannulated screws and hemiarthroplasty [27,28]. Of interest, a high rate of elective implant removal for iliotibial band (ITB) related lateral hip pain has been described by Takigawa et al. using the Targon FN system [23].

The primary aim of this study was to evaluate the number of complications and re-operations following fixation of intracapsular proximal femoral fractures with the Targon FN system and identify risk factors for complications or re-operations. The secondary aim was to identify if lateral prominence of the implant as referenced to the lateral border of the vastus ridge was a specific risk factor for elective plate removal.

2. Materials and Methods

This article was written in accordance with the STROBE-statement [29].

2.1. Patients

This study is a retrospective case series of all consecutive patients older than 18 years treated for an intracapsular proximal femoral fracture with a dynamic locking plate system (Targon® FN) at a single level 1 trauma center in Switzerland between 2010 and 2017. Imaging and patient data were extracted from electronic medical records. All patients received preoperative plain radiographs of the pelvis and a lateral view of the injured hip/proximal femur, intraoperative fluoroscopic images of the operative hip, as well as post-operative plain radiographs of the pelvis and hip. Patients treated for extracapsular fractures with follow up of less than three months or missing imaging and medical data were excluded.

2.2. Implant, Surgical Technique, Rehabilitation and Follow Up

The Targon® FN system (B.Braun AG, Melsungen, Germany) consists of a contoured titanium locking plate, with up to four 6.5 mm telescoping titanium sliding screws (TeleScrews) for fixation into the femoral neck, and two 4.5 mm distal locking screws for fixation to the femoral shaft. The TeleScrews have an integrated telescoping limit of 10–20 mm to prevent the risk of excessive screw back out or collapse (Figure 1).

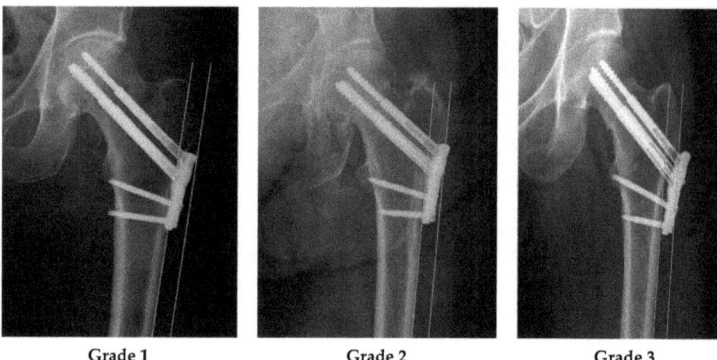

Grade 1　　　　　　　Grade 2　　　　　　　Grade 3

Figure 1. The figure shows the measurement of the plate prominence. One line is parallel to the lateral cortex of the femur, the second line is parallel to the first line and tangential to the distal portion of the trochanter major. In Grade 1 the plate is not cut by the tangential line. In Grade 2, the plate is intersected by the tangential line, in Grade 3 parts of the implant are lateral to the tangential line.

Patients were operated under general anesthesia in the supine position. All patients received a single weight-based dose of cefazolin 30 to 60 min prior to surgery for antibiotic prophylaxis. All procedures were performed under fluoroscopic guidance. For displaced fractures, closed reduction on traction table was first attempted. Open reduction was performed at the discretion of the operating surgeon if an adequate reduction could not be achieved by closed means. For implantation of the Targon implant, a direct lateral approach to the femur was performed by either a trans-vastus approach or by elevation of the vastus lateralis along the posterior boarder of the muscle, depending on the surgeon's preference. The specific surgical technique for the implant system was performed according to the description of Parker MJ et al. [30].

The postoperative rehabilitation protocol consisted of early active-assistive range of motion at the hip joint. Immediate, full weight bearing as tolerated was allowed for stable and non-displaced fractures (Garden I and II) in elderly patients not able to tolerate restricted weightbearing. For patients <65 and those with displaced fractures (Garden III and IV), a 6 to 12-week period of partial weight bearing was advised. All patients used crutches for a minimum of six weeks. At the discretion of the treating surgical team, patients were allowed to wean from crutches if clinical and radiological evaluation showed no secondary displacement and signs of fracture healing at follow-up.

According to our protocol, patients were evaluated postoperatively both radiographically and clinically at six weeks, three months, six months, and one year after surgery. Longer follow up was conducted as clinically necessary, however, if no clinical or radiographic complication had occurred at the 1-year mark, patients were discharged from routine surveillance.

2.3. Data Analysis

Demographic data were collected from of the electronic medical record and operative report including age, sex, smoking status, ASA-Score defined according to the American Society of Anaesthesiologists, dementia (yes/no), diabetes (yes/no), time to operation (from first X-ray until skin incision) (min.), type of reduction (open versus closed versus not necessary), on-call-operation (between 5 pm and 7 am), and number of TeleScrews used (two to four). A diagnosis of osteoporosis was assigned to patients with a T-score <2.5 if a Dual-energy X-ray absorptiometry (DXA) scan was available for review in the clinical record. Table 1 gives an overview of the parameters collected.

Table 1. Baseline Characteristics and Risk Factors (n = 72).

Patient Dependent Factors		Hospital Dependent Factors	
Sex, No. (%)		Time to surgery hours (SD)	
Male	35 (48.6)	Mean	19.99 (20.65)
Female	37 (51.4)	postoperative CCD angle No.	
Age, y		<125	5 (6.94)
Mean (SD)	61.36 (16.35)	125–135	29 (40.28)
Median (range)	60.50 (25–89)	>135	38 (52.78)
Age group, No. (%)		measured TAD (SD)	
<65 y	42 (58.33)	Mean	18.79 (5.05)
≥65 y	30 (41.66)	Reduction No. (%)	
ASA, No. (%)		Open	23 (31.94)
I	10 (13.9)	Closed	29 (40.28)
II	38 (52.8)	Not necessary	20 (27.78)
III	23 (31.9)	Time to full weight bearing weeks No. (%)	
IV	1 (1.4)	Immediately	27 (37.50)
V	0 (0)	6 weeks postoperative	26 (36.11)
Diabetes, No. (%)		10–12 weeks postoperative	19 (26.39)
Type-I	1 (1.4)	Out of office operation No. (%)	
Type-II	3 (4.2)	Yes	33 (45.83)
No	68 (94.4)	No	39 (54.17)
Dementia No. (%)			
Yes	5 (6.9)		
No	67 (93.1)		
Osteoporosis No. (%)			
Yes	10 (86.1)		
No	62 (13.9)		
Smoking status, No. (%)			
Yes	17 (23.6)		
No	55 (76.4)		
AO fracture classification No. (%)			
31-B1	30 (41.7)		
31-B2	35 (48.6)		
31-B3	7 (9.7)		
Garden fracture classification (%)			
Non-displaced	41 (56.9)		
Displaced	31 (43.1)		
Trauma intensity * No. (%)			
Low	51 (70.8)		
High	21 (29.2)		

* Trauma intensity was classified according to ATLS as "low" for fall heights up to 2 meters or speed deltas up to 30 km/h, and as "high" above these values.

Two fellowship-trained trauma surgeons (B.L. and F.B.) evaluated and classified all pre- and postoperative radiographs. The fractures were classified using the AO and Garden fracture classification systems [31,32]. Garden type I and II fractures were categorized as non-displaced and Garden type III and IV as displaced.

The neck-shaft angle was measured on the first postoperative X-ray, one day after surgery using a digital goniometer according to the technique described by Wilson et al. [33].

A neutral neck-shaft angle was assigned to measurements between 120° and 135°, varus if less than 120°, and valgus if more than 135°. The lateral X-ray was used to detect any residual ante- or retro angulation at the fracture site after fixation. The cortical index was also measured on the first postoperative X-ray using a digital ruler, defined as the ratio of cortical width minus endosteal width divided by cortical width at a level of 100 mm below the tip of the lesser trochanter on the anteroposterior radiograph based on the description of Nash et al. [34]. The tip–apex distance was measured between the tip of the nearest TeleScrew to the apex of the femoral head in anteroposterior and axial view referring to the publication by Baumgaertner MR et al. [35]. The result was calibrated by the known lateral diameter (6.5 mm) of the TeleScrew.

If patients had a follow-up of more than 3 months, fracture healing, and no or only category A complication, the position of the lateral plate relative to the vastus ridge was measured and classified using the available intraoperative and postoperative radiographs (Figure 2). The best available anterior posterior hip image was selected based on the profile of the greater trochanter, specifically radiographic overlap of the intertrochanteric ridge and lateral wall of the piriformis fossa [36]. Using this image, a line was created parallel with the lateral cortical border of the femoral diaphysis and tangential to the most lateral border of the vastus ridge. Plates that were positioned medial to this line were classified as Grade 1. Any plate where the most proximal aspect of the plate intersected the line was classified as Grade 2, and plates positioned lateral to the line was classified as Grade 3 (Figure 1).

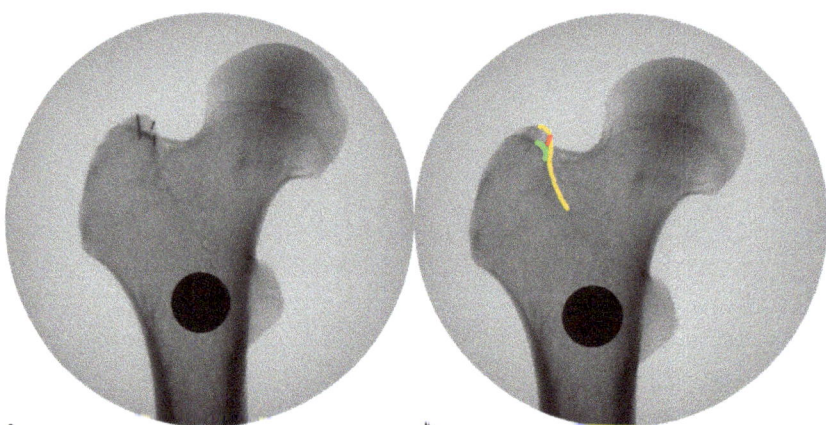

Figure 2. The best available anterior posterior hip image was selected based on the profile of the greater trochanter, specifically radiographic overlap of the intertrochanteric ridge and lateral wall of the piriformis fossa. (**a**): The antero- and postero-superior borders of the greater trochanter overlap in the Cortical Overlap View, this coincides with an overlapping of the easily recognizable intertrochanteric crest and density line of the piriform fossa. (**b**): Yellow marks the intertrochanteric ridge. Green marks the density line of the piriform fossa. Red marks the posterior-superior border of the greater trochanter [36].

The time at which full weight bearing was permitted, as documented by the surgeon in the medical record, was categorized parametrically to either immediately, 6 weeks, 12 weeks, or greater than 12 weeks.

All surgical complications mentioned in the operative report (for example, damage to vascular, nerves, or other structures, additional implants, conversion to arthroplasty) were categorized in this study as intraoperative complications.

Postoperative complications were collected from the medical record and the corresponding x-rays at the post operative follow-up. Only complications directly related to the surgical site were included.

We defined persistent mechanical irritation of the iliotibial band as category A complication. Other complications including plate or screw breakage, screw perforation into the hip joint, secondary loss of reduction (varus deformity with neck-shaft angle <120° or valgus deformity with neck-shaft angle >135°), development of a pathological femoral offset leading to symptomatic femoroactetabular impingement (FAI) and superficial or deep surgical site infections (SSI) were defined as category B. Superficial surgical site infection was defined as an infection of the surgical site involving skin and subcutaneous tissue, occurring within 30 days after surgery. Deep SSI involved soft tissues deep to the subcutaneous tissue and could occur up to one year after surgery [37]. A diagnosis of avascular necrosis was defined by Steinberg stage two or greater on any of the follow up radiographs [38]. Implant failure was defined by any damage of the implants noted on radiographs including breakage of the plate or breakage or loosening of any screws. Non-union was defined if the fracture showed no evidence of bony fusion of at least 2 cortices on conventional X-rays in two planes after 6 months.

Any re-operation at the same surgical site performed after the index operation, including implant removal, was recorded.

2.4. Statistical Analysis

All computations were done with the Statistical Package for Social Sciences (SPSS), version 22 (IBM SPSS Statistics, USA). Continuous data were presented as means with corresponding standard deviation (SD) when normally distributed. In other cases, median with interquartile range (IQR) was used. Categorical variables were presented as counts and corresponding percentages. Differences in continuous variables were analyzed using the independent T-test for normally distributed and Mann–Whitney U test for non-normally distributed variables. Differences in categorical variables were analyzed using the Fisher's exact or Chi-Square test, respectively.

Univariate risk factor analysis was performed using logistic regression and presented as odds ratio's (OR) with corresponding 95% confidence interval (95% CI). $p < 0.05$ was considered statistically significant. No multivariate analysis was possible due to low number of events in the regression model.

3. Results

The study included a total of 83 cases of proximal femur fractures treated with the Targon® FN system between 2010 and 2017. Of these, one was excluded due to a pertrochanteric fracture pattern and ten were excluded due to a follow-up of less than the minimum of three months. Mean follow-up was 19.7 months with a range from 3 to 92 months. A subgroup of 20 patients has a follow-up of less than 12 months. The baseline demographics and risk factors are listed in Table 1.

3.1. Complications and Re-Operations

Forty of seventy-two cases (55.6%) recovered without any category A or B complications and required no unplanned re-operation during the complete follow-up period.

In the 32 remaining cases, at least one complication occurred. The details of these complications can be found in Table 2. Thirty-two cases required one re-operation, and nine patients required more than one re-operation. A total of 46 re-operations were performed. The summary of the re-operations is listed in Table 3.

Table 2. Detailed Listing of Complications with Indication of Underlying Cause. * Percentage of the underlying complication referred to 72 cases. ** Reoperations are indicated by the event that led most likely to the intervention because an associated complication may also lead to a reoperation.

Complications	Cat. A	Cat. B	All	% *	Reoperations **
Hematoma and bleeding					
hematoma	-	1	1	1.4	3
Soft tissue					
tractus irritation	17	-	17	23.6	17
Reduction					
Secondary loss of reduction	-	2	2	2.8	2
Plate and screws					
screw perforation through the cortex of the femoral head	-	5	5	6.9	5
Loosening Tele Screw	-	2	2	2.8	5
Loosening Screw base plate	-	1	1	1.4	1
Osseus disorders					
avascular necrosis of the femoral head	-	4	4	5.6	5
nonunion	-	4	4	5.6	4
postoperative femoroactetabular impingement	-	2	2	2.8	4
Total number	17	21	38	52.8	46

Table 3. The table gives a summary of the resulting 46 re-operations. In the left column, all procedures we performed are listed. If one procedure was performed in one operation the number of cases is found in a diagonal manner (light green fields). Those cases where two procedures were performed in one operation are shown in the lower left of the table (light blue fields). ITB = Ileotibial band.

	Complete Implant Removal	Partial Implant Removal	Total Hip Arthroplasty	Hip Arthroscopy	Revision 90° Blade Plate	Girdlestone Procedure	Revision Total Hip Replacement	Wound Revision	Revision of ITB
Complete implant removal	20								
Partial implant removal		4							
Total hip arthroplasty	6		2						
Monopolar hip arthroplasty	1								
Hip arthroscopy	1			1					
Cement spacer interposition	1								
Removal of cement spacer					1				
Valgus osteotomy with 90° blade plate	1								
Revision 90° blade plate					1				

Table 3. Cont.

	Complete Implant Removal	Partial Implant Removal	Total Hip Arthroplasty	Hip Arthroscopy	Revision 90° Blade Plate	Girdlestone Procedure	Revision Total Hip Replacement	Wound Revision	Revision of ITB
Girdlestone procedure						1			
Exchange of one TeleScrew		1							
Revision total hip replacement							1		
Wound revision								3	
Revision of ITB									1

3.2. Analysis of Risk Factors for Complications

Risk factors for complication (except irritation of the iliotibial band) including ASA-Score, energy of trauma, time to postoperative weight bearing, postoperative caput-collum-diaphyseal (CCD) angle did not show significant differences comparing patients who experienced a complication to patients without complications in univariate analysis. Only age 60 years and younger was observed to be an independent risk for mechanical irritation of the iliotibial band in a univariate logistic regression analysis (OR 8.8, 95% CI 2.3–34.5, $p = 0.001$).

3.3. Analysis of Risk Factors for Re-Operation

Statistical analysis showed that age 60 years and older was significantly related to a lower chance of a second operation (OR 0.25, 95% CI 0.098–0.637, $p = 0.004$). In cases with displaced femoral neck fractures (Garden Type III, IV), there was a significantly higher risk of re-operation (OR = 2.73, 95% CI 1.09–6.83, $p = 0.03$). Moreover, patients that did not reach full weight bearing until after 12 weeks had a significantly higher re-operation rate (OR 3.44, 95% CI 1.07–11.07, $p = 0.04$). Finally, there was a significant correlation between a valgus (>135°) postoperative CCD angle and rate of re-operations (OR 3.11, 95% CI 1.20–8.10, $p = 0.02$). Gender, smoking status, diabetes, osteoporosis, trauma energy did not show a significant association to higher re-operation rates. A complete list of re-operation risk factors is shown in Table 1.

3.4. Plate Position as a Risk Factor for Plate Removal

Fifty-three cases with a follow-up of more than 3 months, fracture union, and no or only category B related complications were analysed to assess the plate position relative to the lateral vastus ridge line described. The plate was classified as Grade 1 in 11 (20.8%) cases, Grade 2 in 36 (69.8%) cases, and Grade 3 in 6 (11.3%) cases. Of the 17 patients who underwent elective plate removal due to lateral hip pain and ITB irritation, 1/11 (9%) was classifed as Grade 1, 14/36 (38%) Grade 2, and 2/6 (33%) grade 3. Relative to Grade 1, the odds ratio for plate removal for Grade 2 was found to be 6.36 (95% CI 0.73–55.30, $p = 0.064$) and 5.00 (95% CI 0.35–71.90, $p = 0.21$) for Grade 3. Although not statistically significant, the data demonstrated a higher risk of plate removal with higher grade of plate position. In all patients, pain resolved after removal of the implant.

4. Discussion

4.1. Key Results

In summary, thirty-four of seventy-two cases (47.2%) treated for an intracapsular femoral neck fracture using the Targon FN system had at least one complication. The most common complication was mechanical irritation of the ITB (23.6%) followed by screw perforation (6.9%), avascular necrosis of the femoral head (5.6%) and non-union (5.6%). Statistical analysis identified patient age 60 years and younger to be an independent risk for mechanical irritation of the iliotibial band. According to statistical analysis, displaced femoral neck fractures (Garden Type III, IV), delayed full weight bearing after 12 months, and a higher postoperative CCD angle (>135°) were significantly associated with re-operations. Although not statistically significant, there is a higher odds ratio for removal of implants in a more laterally prominent position.

4.2. Limitations

The present study has limitations. There was a relatively small number of cases at a single center, with a retrospective study design, and no control or comparison group to other fixation methods. A subgroup of 20 patients has a follow-up of less than 12 months. In this collective, we must assume that we even have underestimated the rate of avascular necrosis, delayed bone healing and irritation of the ITB. Additionally, if patients experienced complication but cared for at outside institutions, the present study would not have captured those events.

Regarding radiographic assessment, there was no standard to ensure the consistency of the AP view acquired used to classify the position of the plate. This was best mitigated by using the best available image of all postoperative and intraoperative views. Furthermore, the technique to determine the TAD was developed for the sliding hip screw with a single screw placed in the femoral head and neck. It is unclear if the concept of TAD applies to an implant consisting of 3 to 4 sliding screws. In the current study the CCD angle was measured on plain ap radiographs. In some cases, it was difficult to define the center of the femoral head for example due to head deformities in cases of osteoarthritis of the hip. Moreover, the definition of the center of the femoral neck was occasionally complicated by posttraumatic deformities. Due to the potential of radiographic technique to confound measurement the clinical significance behind the correlation of high CCD >135° and higher rates of re-operation cannot be made.

4.3. Interpretation

Traditional fixation constructs for intracapsular femoral neck fractures include multiple cannulated screws or sliding hip screw and plate designs. Each of these constructs present unique modes and rates of failure. The literature reports complication rates between 10 and 33% and re-operation rates between 30 and 50% for the treatment of intracapsular proximal femoral fractures using these traditional methods [9–11,19,21,30,39–41]. The Targon FN system was therefore designed to blend the best of both the cannulated screw and sliding hip screw designs by providing multiple smaller diameter screws for fixation into the femoral neck combined with the rigidity of a fixed angled side plate, while allowing for controlled fracture collapse [24].

Literature comparing the Targon FN system to traditional fixation constructs in terms of complication rates is inconsistent. A recent study of two-thousand femoral neck fractures comparing Targon FN to cannulated screws, Alshameeri et al. reported screw cut out in 0.6%, AVN in 7.0% and non-union in 9.5% of all cases treated with the Targon FN system. In cases with displaced femoral neck fractures screw cut out was found in 0.9%, AVN in 8.9% and non-union in 14.4 %. They found the Targon FN System to be associated with lower rates of non-union compared to the cohort treated with cannulated screws. Similar results in smaller cohorts of patients had been previously published by this group. Of note, the authors for these studies included individuals responsible for the design of the Targon FN system implant. At an institution independent from the design institute, Osarumwense et al. reported results in favor of the Targon FN [24]. In this study, a 9% complication rate during a 24 month follow up period. Nearly the same results were published in a study by Sass et al. where they found a 9% rate of complications treated with the Targon FN [42]. In contrast, Griffin et al. found no clinical difference in the risk of revision surgery between the Targon FN (n = 51) and cannulated screw fixation (n = 123) for treatment of intracapsular hip fractures [28]. In this study, 31% of the Targon FN patients and 36% of patients in the cannulated screw group underwent re-operation within 12 months postoperatively.

While in the present study the rate of non-implant associated complication including AVN and non-union is within a similar range as previously reported with this implant, a high rate of implant associated complications due to mechanical irritation of the ITB and lateral hip pain was observed. To our knowledge, there is only one study discussing this finding. Takigawa et al. reported a 10.9% rate of elective implant removal after non-displaced and 48.3% after displaced fractures, for what was reported as discomfort around the implant. In the discussion the authors hypothesized that the size of the Targon FN plate may be too large for the Asian population and could lead to increased irritation of the soft tissue around the plate [23]. The high rate of mechanical irritation in the present study shows that the problem seems not to be limited to an Asian population and potentially due to the position of the plate. Although this study was underpowered to detect a significant correlation between higher grades of implant prominence and rates of implant removal, there was a higher odds ratio of 5 to 6 times for more prominent implant position. Moreover, statistical analysis identified patient age of 60 years and younger to be an independent risk for mechanical irritation of the ITB. We acknowledge that with the use of locking screws in the distal aspect of the plate, there is the possibility of leaving the plate prominent if the surgeon is not conscious to ensure that the plate lies flush against the lateral cortex when applying these locking screws. There could, therefore, be a learning curve associated with this implant resulting in plate prominence that was not accounted for in the current study, but potentially a subject of future study.

The present study aimed to identify risk factors influencing the rate of re-operation. Younger age, fracture dislocation, time to postoperative weight bearing of more than twelve weeks and postoperative caput–collum–diaphyseal (CCD) angle were identified as factors increasing the rate of re-operation. Age less than 60 was the only factor influencing the rate of implant removal. In most other studies the opposite is reported. Carpinetero et al. for example, reported that patients older than 65 years have pre-existing medical comorbidities and thus a higher risk of re-operations and complications (non-unions and avascular necrosis). In our opinion, the higher re-operation rate for younger patients is attributed to a potentially higher activity level of younger patients and resulting in more mechanical irritation around the implant, and possibly more symptomatic than in older, less active patients. We purport that this could lead to a bias toward implant removal and is a reason for younger age as a risk factor for re-operation for implant removal observed in this study.

This study also found a significant correlation between fracture displacement and the likelihood of re-operations. This finding is in line with L.T. Nilsson et al. who reported on a prospective series of femoral neck fractures of 138 patients finding fracture displacement as the only predictive factor of complications [5]. Comparable findings were made by A.Alho et al. in a study with 149 cases of femoral neck fractures. They identified displaced femoral neck fractures to be a risk factor for impaired fracture healing and advocated arthroplasty instead [6]. Parker et al. compared 56 patients with displaced intracapsular fractures randomly treated with hemiarthroplasty or the Targon FN. He found significantly higher reoperation rates and higher postoperative pain in the internal fixation group [43].

Delay to weightbearing beyond 12 weeks was also found as a risk fractor for re-operation. In fact, recent studies recommend an early transition to full weight bearing [8,44]. A study by Kolaczko et al. showed that limiting weight bearing for more than 8 weeks may negatively affect bone healing [44]. In turn, this could lead to prolonged higher loads on the implant and thus promote implant failure. However, bias toward cautious aftercare may be influenced by many factors including the experience of the treating surgeon, patient age, general medical condition of the patient, a somewhat less than perfect reduction or implant position. Therefore, this finding may be a surrogate parameter for other risk factors rather than a risk factor on its own.

5. Conclusions

In summary, there is a high complication rate for patients treated for intracapsular femoral neck fracture using the Targon FN system. The most common complication was mechanical irritation of the iliotibial band around the implant. Age 60 years and younger was an independent risk factor for ITB irritation requiring plate removal. We hypothesize this is associated with lateral plate prominence and higher activity levels in younger patients. Statistical analysis showed that patient age, fracture dislocation, time to postoperative full weight bearing were risk factors for re-operation. In our opinion, if the Targon FN system is utilized, plate position should be as flush as possible to avoid mechanical irritation of the ITB.

Author Contributions: Conceptualization, E.K., J.G. and B.-C.L.; methodology, E.K., J.G. and B.-C.L.; software, E.K., J.G.; validation, E.K., J.G. and B.-C.L.; formal analysis, E.K., J.G., B.J.M.v.d.W. and B.-C.L.; investigation, E.K., J.G.; resources, E.K., J.G.; data curation, E.K., J.G.; writing—original draft preparation, E.K., J.G.; writing—review and editing, D.E.D., B.J.M.v.d.W., M.K.; R.B.; F.J.P.B.; visualization, E.K.; supervision, B.-C.L.; project administration, B.-C.L. All authors have read and agreed to the published version of the manuscript.

Funding: This research received no external funding.

Institutional Review Board Statement: The study was conducted in accordance with the Declaration of Helsinki.

Informed Consent Statement: Informed consent was obtained from all subjects involved in the study.

Data Availability Statement: Data supporting reported results are stored by the corresponding author.

Conflicts of Interest: The authors declare no conflict of interest.

References

1. Parker, M.J.; Cawley, S. Cemented or uncemented hemiarthroplasty for displaced intracapsular fractures of the hip: A randomized trial of 400 patients. *Bone Jt. J.* **2019**, *102-B*, 11–16. [CrossRef] [PubMed]
2. Stöckle, U.; Lucke, M.; Haas, N.P. Der Oberschenkelhalsbruch. *Dtsch. Arztebl.* **2005**, *102*, 3426–3434.
3. Knobe, M.; Siebert, C.H. Hüftgelenknahe Frakturen im hohen Lebensalter. *Orthopäde* **2014**, *43*, 314–324. [CrossRef] [PubMed]
4. Blomfeldt, R.; Törnkvist, H.; Ponzer, S.; Söderqvist, A.; Tidermark, J. Comparison of Internal Fixation with Total Hip Replacement for Displaced Femoral Neck Fractures: Randomized, Controlled Trial Performed at Four Years. *JBJS* **2005**, *87*, 1680–1688. [CrossRef]
5. Nilsson, L.T.; Johansson, Å.; Strömqvist, B. Factors predicting healing complications in femoral neck fractures: 138 patients followed for 2 years. *Acta Orthop. Scand.* **1993**, *64*, 175–177. [CrossRef] [PubMed]
6. Alho, A.; Benterud, J.G.; Rønningen, H.; Høiseth, A. Prediction of disturbed healing in femoral neck fracture. *Acta Orthop. Scand.* **1992**, *63*, 639–644. [CrossRef]
7. Dolatowski, F.C.; Frihagen, F.; Bartels, S.; Opland, V.; Benth, J.Š.; Talsnes, O.; Hoelsbrekken, S.E.; Utvåg, S.E. Screw Fixation Versus Hemiarthroplasty for Nondisplaced Femoral Neck Fractures in Elderly Patients: A Multicenter Randomized Controlled Trial. *J. Bone Joint Surg. Am.* **2019**, *101*, 136–144. [CrossRef]
8. Maffulli, N.; Aicale, R. Proximal Femoral Fractures in the Elderly: A Few Things to Know, and Some to Forget. *Medicina Mex* **2022**, *58*, 1314. [CrossRef]
9. Ly, T.; Swiontkowski, M. Treatment of femoral neck fractures in young adults. *J. Bone Jt. Surg. Am.* **2008**, *90*, 2254–2266. [CrossRef]
10. Parker, M.J.; Raghavan, R.; Gurusamy, K. Incidence of fracture-healing complications after femoral neck fractures. *Clin. Orthop.* **2007**, *458*, 175–179. [CrossRef]
11. Lu-Yao, G.L.; Keller, R.B.; Littenberg, B.; Wennberg, J.E. Outcomes after displaced fractures of the femoral neck. A meta-analysis of one hundred and six published reports. *J. Bone Jt. Surg.—Ser. A* **1994**, *76*, 15–25. [CrossRef] [PubMed]
12. Knobe, M.; Altgassen, S.; Maier, K.-J.; Gradl-Dietsch, G.; Kaczmarek, C.; Nebelung, S.; Klos, K.; Kim, B.; Gueorguiev, B.; Horst, K.; et al. Screw-blade fixation systems in Pauwels three femoral neck fractures: A biomechanical evaluation. *Int. Orthop.* **2018**, *42*, 409–418. [CrossRef] [PubMed]

13. Hsueh, K.-K.; Fang, C.-K.; Chen, C.-M.; Su, Y.-P.; Wu, H.-F.; Chiu, F.-Y. Risk factors in cutout of sliding hip screw in intertrochanteric fractures: An evaluation of 937 patients. *Int. Orthop.* **2010**, *34*, 1273–1276. [CrossRef] [PubMed]
14. Song, H.K.; Choi, H.J.; Yang, K.H. Risk factors of avascular necrosis of the femoral head and fixation failure in patients with valgus angulated femoral neck fractures over the age of 50 years. *Injury* **2016**, *47*, 2743–2748. [CrossRef] [PubMed]
15. Van Embden, D.; Roukema, G.R.; Rhemrev, S.J.; Genelin, F.; Meylaerts, S.A.G. The Pauwels classification for intracapsular hip fractures: Is it reliable? *Injury* **2011**, *42*, 1238–1240. [CrossRef] [PubMed]
16. Caviglia, H.A.; Quintana Osorio, P.; Comando, D. Classification and diagnosis of intracapsular fractures of the proximal femur. *Clin. Orthop.* **2002**, *399*, 17–27. [CrossRef] [PubMed]
17. Hoshino, C.M.; O'Toole, R.V. Fixed angle devices versus multiple cancellous screws: What does the evidence tell us? *Injury* **2015**, *46*, 474–477. [CrossRef]
18. Linde, F.; Andersen, E.; Hvass, I.; Madsen, F.; Pallesen, R. Avascular femoral head necrosis following fracture fixation. *Injury* **1986**, *17*, 159–163. [CrossRef]
19. Nauth, A.; Creek, A.T.; Zellar, A.; Lawendy, A.R.; Dowrick, A.; Gupta, A.; Dadi, A.; van Kampen, A.; Yee, A.; de Vries, A.C.; et al. Fracture fixation in the operative management of hip fractures (FAITH): An international, multicentre, randomised controlled trial. *Lancet* **2017**, *389*, 1519–1527. [CrossRef]
20. Thein, R.; Herman, A.; Kedem, P.; Chechik, A.; Shazar, N. Osteosynthesis of unstable intracapsular femoral neck fracture by dynamic locking plate or screw fixation: Early results. *J. Orthop. Trauma* **2014**, *28*, 70–76. [CrossRef]
21. Parker, M.; Cawley, S.; Palial, V. Internal fixation of intracapsular fractures of the hip using a dynamic locking plate: Two-year follow-up of 320 patients. *Bone Jt. J.* **2013**, *95*, 1402–1405. [CrossRef] [PubMed]
22. Körver, R.J.P.; Wieland, A.W.J.; Kaarsemaker, S.; Nieuwenhuis, J.J.; Janzing, H.M.J. Clinical experience, primary results and pitfalls in the treatment of intracapsular hip fractures with the Targon® FN locking plate. *Injury* **2013**, *44*, 1926–1929. [CrossRef] [PubMed]
23. Takigawa, N.; Yasui, K.; Eshiro, H.; Moriuchi, H.; Abe, M.; Tsujinaka, S.; Kinoshita, M. Clinical results of surgical treatment for femoral neck fractures with the Targon® FN. *Injury* **2016**, *47*, S44–S48. [CrossRef] [PubMed]
24. Osarumwense, D.; Tissingh, E.; Wartenberg, K.; Aggarwal, S.; Ismail, F.; Orakwe, S.; Khan, F. The targon FN system for the management of intracapsular neck of femur fractures: Minimum 2-year experience and outcome in an independent hospital. *CiOS Clin. Orthop. Surg.* **2015**, *7*, 22–28. [CrossRef] [PubMed]
25. Alshameeri, Z.; Elbashir, M.; Parker, M.J. The outcome of intracapsular hip fracture fixation using the Targon Femoral Neck (TFN) locking plate system or cannulated cancellous screws: A comparative study involving 2004 patients. *Injury* **2017**, *48*, 2555–2562. [CrossRef] [PubMed]
26. Hou, X.; Shi, G.; Zhang, Y.; Xing, B.; Xu, D. Comparison between Three Cannulated Screws and Targon Locking Plate for Displaced Intracapsular Hip Fracture: A Retrospective Stud. *Res. Sq.* **2022**, preprint. [CrossRef]
27. Parker, M.J.; Pryor, G.; Gurusamy, K. Hemiarthroplasty versus internal fixation for displaced intracapsular hip fractures: A long-term follow-up of a randomised trial. *Injury* **2010**, *41*, 370–373. [CrossRef]
28. Griffin, X.L.; Parsons, N.; Achten, J.; Costa, M.L. The Targon Femoral Neck hip screw versus cannulated screws for internal fixation of intracapsular fractures of the hip. *Bone. Jt. J.* **2014**, *96-B*, 652–657. [CrossRef]
29. von Elm, E.; Altman, D.G.; Egger, M.; Pocock, S.J.; Gøtzsche, P.C.; Vandenbroucke, J.P. The strengthening the reporting of observational studies in epidemiology (STROBE) statement: Guidelines for reporting observational studies. *Int. J. Surg.* **2014**, *12*, 1495–1499. [CrossRef]
30. Parker, M.J.; Stedtfeld, H.-W. Internal fixation of intracapsular hip fractures with a dynamic locking plate: Initial experience and results for 83 patients treated with a new implant. *Injury* **2010**, *41*, 348–351. [CrossRef]
31. Garden, R.S. Low-Angle Fixation in Fractures of the Femoral Neck. *Bone Jt. J.* **1961**, *43-B*, 647–663. [CrossRef]
32. Müller, M.E.; Koch, P.; Nazarian, S.; Schatzker, J. *The Comprehensive Classification of Fractures of Long Bones*; Springer: Berlin/Heidelberg, Germany, 1990. [CrossRef]
33. Wilson, J.D.; Eardley, W.; Odak, S.; Jennings, A. To what degree is digital imaging reliable? Validation of femoral neck shaft angle measurement in the era of picture archiving and communication systems. *Br. J. Radiol.* **2011**, *84*, 375–379. [CrossRef]
34. Nash, W.; Harris, A. The Dorr type and cortical thickness index of the proximal femur for predicting peri-operative complications during hemiarthroplasty. *J. Orthop. Surg.* **2014**, *22*, 92–95. [CrossRef] [PubMed]
35. Baumgaertner, M.R.; Curtin, S.L.; Lindskog, D.M.; Keggi, J.M. The value of the tip-apex distance in predicting failure of fixation of peritrochanteric fractures of the hip. *J. Bone Jt. Surg.* **1995**, *77*, 1058–1064. [CrossRef] [PubMed]
36. Link, B.-C.; van Veelen, N.M.; Boernert, K.; Kittithamvongs, P.; Beeres, F.J.P.; de Boer, H.H.; Migliorini, F.; Nebelung, S.; Knobe, M.; Ruchholtz, S.; et al. The radiographic relationship between the cortical overlap view (COV) and the tip of the greater trochanter. *Sci. Rep.* **2021**, *11*, 18404. [CrossRef]
37. Horan, T.C.; Gaynes, R.P.; Martone, W.J.; Jarvis, W.R.; Emori, T.G. CDC Definitions of Nosocomial Surgical Site Infections, 1992, A Modification of CDC Definitions of Surgical Wound Infections. *Infect. Control Hosp. Epidemiol.* **1992**, *13*, 606–608. [CrossRef] [PubMed]
38. Steinberg, M.E.; Hayken, G.D.; Steinberg, D.R. A quantitative system for staging avascular necrosis. *J. Bone Jt. Surg. Br.* **1995**, *77*, 34–41. [CrossRef]

39. Parker Martyn, J.; Gurusamy Kurinchi, S. Internal fixation implants for intracapsular hip fractures in adults. *Cochrane Database Syst. Rev.* **2011**, *4*, 1465–1858. [CrossRef]
40. Loizou, C.L.; Parker, M.J. Avascular necrosis after internal fixation of intracapsular hip fractures; a study of the outcome for 1023 patients. *Injury* **2009**, *40*, 1143–1146. [CrossRef]
41. Damany, D.S.; Parker, M.J.; Chojnowski, A. Complications after intracapsular hip fractures in young adults: A meta-analysis of 18 published studies involving 564 fractures. *Injury* **2005**, *36*, 131–141. [CrossRef]
42. Saß, M.; Mittlmeier, T. Joint-preserving treatment of medial femoral neck fractures with an angular stable implant. *Oper. Orthop. Traumatol.* **2016**, *28*, 291–308. [CrossRef] [PubMed]
43. Parker, M.J. Hemiarthroplasty versus internal fixation for displaced intracapsular fractures of the hip in elderly men. *Bone Jt. J.* **2015**, *97-B*, 992–996. [CrossRef] [PubMed]
44. Kolaczko, J.G.; McMellen, C.J.; Magister, S.J.; Wetzel, R.J. Comparison of time to healing and major complications after surgical fixation of nondisplaced femoral neck stress fractures: A systematic review. *Injury* **2021**, *52*, 647–652. [CrossRef] [PubMed]

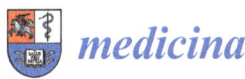

Article

The Influence of a Modified 3rd Generation Cementation Technique and Vaccum Mixing of Bone Cement on the Bone Cement Implantation Syndrome (BCIS) in Geriatric Patients with Cemented Hemiarthroplasty for Femoral Neck Fractures

Ulf Bökeler [1,*], Alissa Bühler [1], Daphne Eschbach [2], Christoph Ilies [3], Ulrich Liener [1] and Tom Knauf [2]

1. Department for Orthopaedics and Trauma Surgery, Marienhospital Stuttgart Böheimstrasse 37, 70199 Stuttgart, Germany
2. Center for Orthopaedics and Trauma Surgery, University Hospital Giessen and Marburg, 35039 Marburg, Germany
3. Department for Anesthesia and Intensive Care, Marienhospital Stuttgart, 70199 Stuttgart, Germany
* Correspondence: ulfwilhelm.boekeler@vinzenz.de; Tel.: +49-711-6489-2203

Abstract: *Background and Objectives:* Cemented hemi arthroplasty is a common and effective procedure performed to treat femoral neck fractures in elderly patients. The bone cement implantation syndrome (BCIS) is a severe and potentially fatal complication which can be associated with the implantation of a hip prosthesis. The aim of this study was to investigate the influence of a modified cementing technique on the incidence of BCIS. *Material and Methods:* The clinical data of patients which were treated with a cemented hip arthroplasty after the introduction of the modified 3rd generation cementing technique were compared with a matched group of patients who were treated with a 2nd generation cementing technique. The anesthesia charts for all patients were reviewed for the relevant parameters before, during and after cementation. Each patient was classified as having no BCIS (grade 0) or BCIS grade 1,2, or 3 depending on the severity of hypotension, hypoxia loss of consciousness. *Results:* A total of 92 patients with complete data sets could be included in the study. The mean age was 83 years. 43 patients (Group A) were treated with a 2nd and 49 patients (Group B) with a 3rd generation cementing technique. The incidence of BCIS grade 1,2, and 3 was significantly higher ($p = 0{,}036$) in group A (n = 25; 58%) compared to group B (n = 17; 35%). Early mortality was higher in group A (n = 4) compared to group B (n = 0). *Conclusions:* BCIS is a potentially severe complication with a significant impact on early mortality following cemented hemiarthroplasty of the hip for the treatment of proximal femur fracture. Using a modified 3rd generation cementing technique, it is possible to significantly reduce the incidence of BCIS and its associated mortality.

Keywords: bone cement implantation syndrome; cementation technique; femoral neck fracture; hip hemiarthroplasty

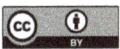

1. Introduction

Femoral neck fractures are common injuries in elderly patients. Despite advances in the medical and surgical management, these injuries are still associated with a peri- and postoperative 30-day mortality of up to 10% [1]. Despite a short modulation of incidence during the COVID epidemic, the total number of fractures is expected to rise significantly in the next decade [2]. In elderly, less mobile patients cemented hemiarthroplasty is the currently recommended treatment of choice for displaced femoral fractures [3]. Although associated with a longer operation time, cemented hemiarthroplasty leads to faster recovery, less pain and better functional results than uncemented fixation of the femoral stem [4–8].

Despite these superior clinical results and a lower revision rate of cemented stems [4–7] the use of cement still remains controversial [9–11], because cemented hip arthroplasty can be associated with the development of bone cement implantation syndrome (BCIS).

First described by Donaldson 2009 it is a potentially fatal complication characterized by transient oxygen desaturation, hypotension, acute increase in pulmonary arterial resistance which in severe cases can lead to right ventricular and subsequent life-threatening cardiovascular failure requiring cardiopulmonary resuscitation [12–14]. The occurrence of BCIS has resulted in an extensive debate about the fixation of the femoral stem and considerable variation in the practice. Although there is an abundance of literature comparing cemented to uncemented arthroplasty for the treatment of proximal femur fracture [5,7,8,10,15–17] there is a scarcity of data available for surgical measures to prevent BCIS. So far, only a single prospective randomized interventional study has analyzed the impact of a modified implantation technique on the incidence and severity of BCIS [18].

The aim of the present study was therefore to investigate the influence of a comprehensive cementing technique on the development of BCIS in a geriatric patient population with hip fractures treated with cemented hemi arthroplasty.

2. Material and Methods

After approval by the Institutional review Board, we included all patients into this retrospective study that received a primary cemented hemiarthroplasty due to a femoral neck fracture between January 2007 and December 2015. Between January 2007 and July 2010, a 2nd generation cementing technology was used. Between January 2014 and December 2015, we used a third generation cementing technology. The data collected (from the time of admission to discharge) was extracted from the patient file, the surgical reports and the anesthesia protocols. The following patient characteristics were recorded: age, sex and place of residence. Comorbidities and the severity of pre-existing conditions were determined using the Charlson Comorbidity Index (CCI) [19] and the American Society of Anesthesiologists (ASA) risk classification [20]. In addition, time to surgery, duration of the surgery, type of anesthesia, intraoperative blood pressure, oxygen saturation and adverse perioperative cardiovascular reactions, length of stay, and peri- and postoperative complications were assessed.

The Bone Cement Implantation Syndrome Grades were classified according to Donaldson et al. [12] (Table 1).

Table 1. Classification Bone Cement Implantation Syndrome.

Grade 1	moderate hypoxia (arterial oxygen saturation < 94%) or hypotension (a decrease in systolic arterial pressure (SAP) > 20%)
Grade 2	severe hypoxia (arterial oxygen saturation < 88%) or hypotension (a decrease in SAP > 40%) or unexpected loss of consciousness
Grade 3	cardiovascular collapse requiring cardiopulmonary resuscitation

Initially, 203 patients with complete data sets were included. Because of inconsistent documentation of the exact time, 111 patients had to be excluded. Depending on the technique of cementation, these patients were divided in two groups. Group A consists of patients who were operated with the second-generation cementing technology, whereas group B had been operated on with a modified third generation cementing technology (Figure 1).

2.1. Surgical Technique

All procedures were performed under general anesthesia and monitored by electrocardigram, non-invasive blood pressure management and pulse oximetry. In patients with severe concomitant medical conditions, the monitoring was extended by invasive blood pressure measurement and measurement of the central venous pressure. Prior to cement implantation, the patients were preoxygenated with an FiO2 of 1.0.

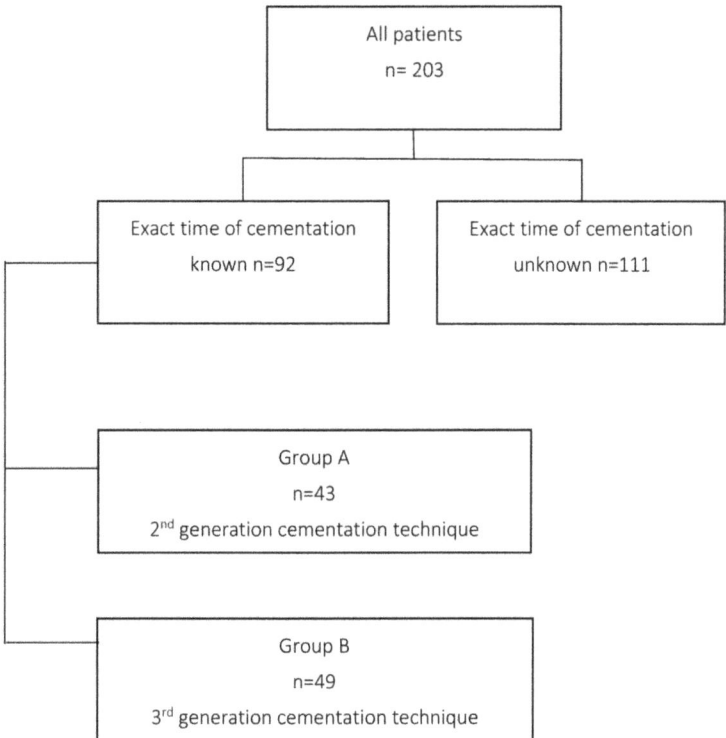

Figure 1. Flowchart.

In all patients an appropriately sized stem (Bicontact®, Aesculap, Tuttlingen, Germany) was cemented with Palacos® (Heraeus Medical, Wehrheim, Germany) through an anterolateral approach in a supine position.

In patients of group A, the 2nd generation cementing technique was used: After femoral canal preparation, a distal cement restrictor was inserted. Then cement was mixed in open atmosphere by hand in an open plastic bowl supplied by the cement manufacturer.

The bone bed was rinsed with a syringe. The cement was applied in a retrograde fashion with the cement gun and the stem was inserted.

In patients of group B, a modified 3rd generation cementing technique was used: After femoral canal preparation, a distal cement restrictor was inserted. The bone bed was thoroughly cleaned with a jet lavage. Cement (Palacos® Heraeus Medical) was mixed with a vacuum mixing system provided by the cement manufacturer (Palamix® Heraeus Medical). Residual blood was removed by lavaging the femoral canal with the jet lavage (Interpulse® Stryker, Kalamazoo, MI, USA). The cement was inserted in a retrograde fashion with a cement gun without a femoral pressurizer.

2.2. Statistical Analysis

Statistical analysis was carried out with the SPSS Statistic Program (Version 23, SPSS Inc., Chicago, IL, USA). The level of significance was on $\alpha = 0.05$ two sided fixed. For comparison of the relative frequency of the BCIS the Chi Quadrat Test, two unpaired tests were used. Further significance analysis of the study results was taken through for nominal variables by the Chi Quadrat Test, for ordinal variables with the Mann-Whitney-U-Tests. For not normally distributed variables, the median was determined.

3. Results

The average age of the 92 patients was 83 years (58–99 years.), 65 were female (71%), and 27 (29%) male (Table 2). The demographic, medical and surgery related date are shown in Table 1. There was no significant difference in the demographic data of the patients.

Table 2. Patients characteristics, * $p < 0.05$ (significant).

	Group A	Group B
Age (median)	81	84
Gender n (%)		
- Female	30 (70%)	35 (71%)
- Male	13 (30%)	14 (29%)
Residence n (%)		
- Independent	22 (51%)	30 61%)
- Nursing home	9 (21%)	16 (33%)
- Hospital or rehab clinic	5 (12%)	2 (4%)
- Unknown	7 (16%)	1 (2%)
ASA Grade n (%)		
- ASA 1	0	0
- ASA 2	7 (16%)	14 (29%)
- ASA 3	30 (70%)	33 (67%)
- ASA 4	6 (14%)	2 (4%)
CCI (median)	3	3
Time to surgery in hours n (%)		
- <24	28 (65%) *	42 (86%) *
- 24–48	9 (21%)	5 (11%)
- 48–72	2 (5%)	2 (4%)
- >72	4 (9%)	0

The proportioning of the patients in the Charlson Comorbidity Index showed a variation in total from 0–9 points with a median of 3 points. There was no difference in the variation of the CCI in between the groups with a median of 3 in both groups.

The majority of the patients (91%) were operated on in the first 48 h following admission. In group B significantly more patients were operated within the first 24 h after admission (Table 2).

The statistical analysis of age, ASA score, CCI and duration of the operation did not reveal a statistical difference between group A and B.

3.1. Occurrence of BCIS

42 patients (46%) developed a BCIS. The BCIS occurred significantly ($p = 0.036$) more frequently in Group A (2nd generation cementing technique) (n = 25, 58%) than in Group B (3rd generation cementing technique) (n = 17, 35%). In addition, when BCIS occurred it was more pronounced in patients of Group A (Figure 2).

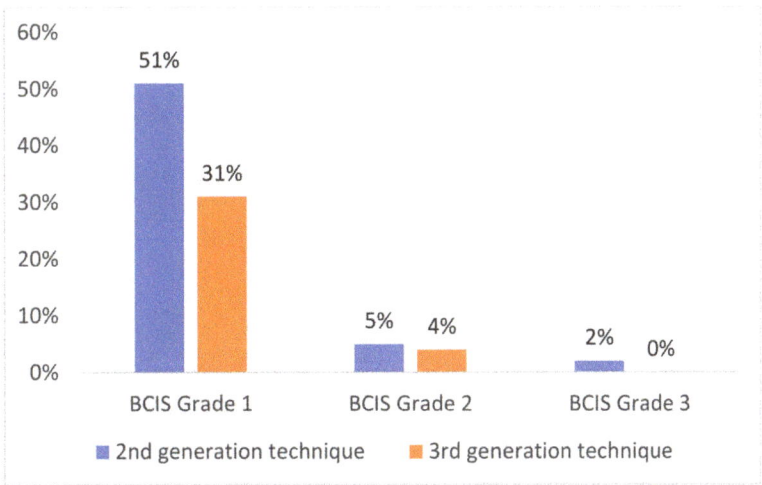

Figure 2. Severity of BCIS in 2nd and 3rd generation technique.

3.2. Complications and Mortality

The postoperative complication rate of all patients was 32% (n = 29). Patients of Group A showed a slightly higher rate of complications (n = 15 (35%)) than patients of Group B (n = 14 (29%)), without being statistically significant. The majority of the complication were medical complications and not directly related to the surgery itself (Table 3).

Table 3. Overview of complications.

Postoperative Complications	Group A n (%)	Group B n (%)
Overall complications	15 (35%)	14 (29%)
Hip Dislocation	0	1 (2%)
Surgical Site Infection	3 (7%)	2 (4%)
Haematoma	2 (5%)	0
Cardiopulmonary	5 (12%)	5 (10%)
Pulmonary embolism	0	0
Renal failure	0	2 (4%)
Delirium	1 (2%)	4 (8%)
Mortality	4 (10%)	0

There were four perioperative deaths in Group A and none in Group B. Three of the four patients that died suffered a BCIS. An overview of al complications distributed to the different groups is shown in Table 3.

The likelihood of complications was increased if BCIS occurred with 15 complications (36%) in BCIS positive group compared to 14 complications (28%) in the BCIS negative group (Table 4).

Table 4. Postoperative Complications in BCIS positive and negative patients.

Postoperative Complications	BCIS Positive	BCIS Negative
	n (%)	n (%)
Number of patients	42 (100%)	50 (100%)
Overall complications	15 (36%)	14 (28%)
Hip Dislocation	0	1 (2%)
Infection	3 (7%)	2 (4%)
Hematoma	1 (2%)	1 (2%)
Cardiopulmonary	5 (12%)	5 (10%)
Pulmonary embolism	0	0
Renal failure	1 (2%)	1 (2%)
Delir	2 (5%)	3 (6%)
Death	3 (7%)	1 (2%)

4. Discussion

Analysis of large registries has demonstrated a high revision rate following uncemented arthroplasty for hip fracture due to periprosthetic femur fractures in [7,21]. Because of the aforementioned scientific data, the NICE guidelines and the National Hip Fracture Data Base in Great Britain use cemented fixation of the femoral component as a marker of quality for patients with femoral neck fractures [22]. However cemented arthroplasty can be associated with Bone Cement Implantation Syndrome (BCIS). First described and classified by Donaldson, it has a wide spectrum of clinical features that range from transient oxygen desaturation, hypotension to cardiovascular collapse requiring cardiopulmonary resuscitation [12]. The clinical features typically occur at a time of cementation but can also occur at the insertion of an uncemented stem.

The incidence of BCIS varies between 19% and 53% [18,23,24]. It is likely that the real incidence is higher because mild reactions with a blood pressure drop below 20% are not classified as BCIS. The distribution of the severity of BCIS in our study is comparable to the data from Olsen et al. [25]. The high incidences of BCIS do document that it is a potential problem for patients suffering from a proximal femur fracture. A recent analysis documented a trend towards excess mortality in a subgroup of ASA class IV patients [26]. Therefore, identification of frail the patients with poor cardiorespiratory reserves and who are most likely to be affected is paramount in the prevention of BCIS.

Since in-hospital mortality is significantly increased if BCIS occurs, several anesthesiology and surgical measures have been recommended to decrease the incidence of BCIS [23]. The surgical measures include the routine insertion of intramedullary plugs, the placement of medullary drains during cement insertion or alternatively a femoral bore hole and the placement of the patients in a lateral decubitus position in the case of pulmonary disease [18,27]. These surgical recommendations are rather based on assumptions deducted from the analysis on cemented vs. uncemented arthroplasties and not from results of interventional studies.

So far, only a single study has investigated the impact of a modified cementing technique on the development of BCIS. In a prospective randomized study on 72 patients, Leidinger et al. were able to demonstrate a significant reduction in mortality from 14% in the control group and 3% in the group where the bone cement was prepared with a vacuum mixing system. In addition, the rate of echocardiographically diagnosed pulmonary embolism and circulatory insufficiency was significantly decreased. Unfortunately, they did not grade the severity of the BCIS according to Donaldson; therefore, a direct comparison with our study is not possible [18]. In contrast to our study, they did not use an intramedullary plug and pulsatile lavage before implanting the stem. Our study is the first to investigate the impact of a modified 3rd generation cementing technique on the development of BCIS. We were able to demonstrate a significant reduction in the incidence of BCIS when a modified 3rd generation cementation technique was used (35% 3rd generation vs. 58% 2nd generation cementation technique). The 3rd generation cementing technique aims to improve the inter interlock of cement through thorough bone bed preparation with a pulsatile lavage, use of a distal cement restrictor, retrograde cement application and preparation of cement in a vacuum and femoral pressurization [28].

Bone cement consists of two components. Pre- polymerized polymethyl methacrylate (PMMA) which is present as white powder and the liquid monomer of methyl methacrylate (MMA). When mixing the substances, a catalyst initiates the polymerization of the monomer fluid and the PMMA "pearls" are entrapped within the polymerized monomer.

There is compelling evidence that bone cement is an independent risk factor in the development of BCIS. Christie et al. were able to show that the cemented arthroplasty caused greater and more prolonged embolic cascades than did uncemented arthroplasty [29]. The exact mechanism of this cement mediated pulmonary embolism remains unclear because monomer concentrations in the circulation are very low [30].

Vacuum preparation of cement has been shown to reduce micro and macro pores, resulting in improved strength with a lower risk of aseptic loosening [30]. In addition, vacuum bone cement mixing systems have been shown to significantly remove monomer fumes [31]. It has been hypothesized that monomer-mediated vasoconstriction and mediator release, complement activation and endothelial damage caused by cement particles induce vasoconstriction and pulmonary vascular resistance [12,30]. Given the results of our study and that of Leidinger et al. it is highly likely that the removal of monomer fumes has a significant clinical impact because the vacuum cementing technique significantly reduced the incidence of BCIS.

Although the pathophysiology of BCIS still is not completely understood, there is evidence that pulmonary embolism plays a key role in the etiology of BCIS. Embolic material can be detected in 60% of patients with cemented hip replacement compared to 6% of patients with uncemented hip replacement [32]. In addition, Leidinger et al. were able to detect intra pulmonary thrombotic material in all patients with BCIS that were resuscitated [18].

The use of a pulsatile lavage removes debris caused by femoral canal preparation and fatty marrow particles facilitating cement interdigitation. Given the pathophysiology of BCIS, it is highly likely that thorough jet lavage also reduced the number of intramedullary particles that could dislodge into the systemic circulation, resulting in reduced histamine release, complement activation and emboli formation. In addition to pulsatile lavage, we consistently used a distal cement restrictor (plug) in all patients. In contrast to Weingärtner et al., who have advocated against a medullary plug, we believe that placing a medullary plug does reduce the intramedullary volume by creating a "cement compartment" thereby reducing the overall number of intramedullary particles that can potentially dislodge into the circulation. In addition, we further reduced the intramedullary pressure by not using a proximal pressurization device. We were able to show that the addition of pulsatile lavage and a distal cement restrictor to vacuum cementing technique not only reduces the perioperative mortality, but also decreases the incidence of BCIS.

The total complication rate in our study was 32%, which is comparable to other series [10,15], while implant associated complications occurred less frequently than in the literature with 7 % [11,15]. BCIS positive patients showed an increased number of postoperative complications compared to patients who did not develop a BCIS, without being statistically significant. In our study, the incidence of BCIS did not increase with advancing age. This unexcepted finding is difficult to explain because patient related risk factors for the development for BCIS, like age [23], cardiovascular diseases [18,23,33,34] and malignant diseases [35,36] are well described and influence the development and characteristic of a BCIS. Accordingly, in our study, we were not able to determine any significant influence of the ASA score of the patients on developing a BCIS. Although there was an increased incidence of BCIS in patients with ASA 3, we could not find any significance in contrast to the study of Weingärtner et al., which identified the ASA Score as an independent risk factor [23]. Other risk factors, described in the literature are COPD and the long-term medication with warfarin or diuretics [24].

The study has several limitations. It is a retrospective study. Not all data could be collected completely, also the documentation accuracy varied. In several cases, the time of the application of cement was not noted in the anaestheological protocol, therefore these patients could not be included in the study. The sample size of both groups was different. However, a comparative analysis of the patients did not reveal any statistically significant differences in the demographic and outcome parameters of the sample subgroups.

5. Conclusions

Although associated with a longer operation time, treatment of proximal femur fractures with cemented hemi or total arthroplasty leads to better functional results and a lower reoperation rate than uncemented fixation of the femoral stem. Nevertheless, BCIS is a potentially severe complication, with a significant impact on early mortality. In our study, we were able to show that using a modified 3rd generation cementing technique, it is possible to significantly reduce the incidence of BCIS and therefore its associated mortality. Further studies are warranted to elucidate the pathophysiology of BCIS.

A rapid response report concerning the perioperative mortality following cemented arthroplasty for hip fractures by the National Patient Safety Agency in Great Britain in 2009 has led to an extensive analysis of a large number of patients from national registries. These revealed an increase in deaths following cemented arthroplasty in the first 24 h following surgery compared to uncemented arthroplasty [37]. However, an analysis of 16.496 patients from British Nation Hip Fracture Data Base documented significantly lower deaths at discharge in patients with cemented arthroplasty [22]. The findings that cemented arthroplasty does not increase the perioperative mortality has been confirmed by a recent meta-analysis [38].

In a recent study by Weingärtner et al. on a comparable patient population using vacuum mixing system, 37% of patients developed BCIS [23]. The authors investigated risk factors for the development of BCIS were able to identify age, ASA score and, as the only modifiable parameter, the (non) placement of a distal bore hole as significant risk factors. It is noteworthy that only 28% of the patients did receive a bore hole.

This tendency towards a higher complication rate is clearer presented by the work of Weingärtner et al. [23] who showed a significantly higher rate of cardiovascular complications and a higher in-hospital mortality rate for BCIS positive patients. Work by Olsen et al. demonstrated that with higher BCIS stages, the one year mortality rate is increasing [25].

Author Contributions: Conceptualization, U.B., U.L. and T.K.; methodology, U.B., A.B. and U.L.; software, A.B.; validation, U.B., A.B. and U.L. formal analysis, U.B. and T.K.; investigation, U.B., A.B. and U.L.; resources, U.B. and U.L.; data curation, U.B., A.B.; writing—original draft preparation, U.B., U.L. and T.K.; writing—review and editing, All authors; visualization, U.B. and A.B.; supervision, D.E. and C.I. All authors have read and agreed to the published version of the manuscript.

Funding: This research received no external funding.

Institutional Review Board Statement: The study was conducted according to the guidelines of the Declaration of Helsinki and approved by the Institutional Review Board (or Ethics Committee) of Baden Württemberg, Germany on the 14 December 2016.

Informed Consent Statement: Patient consent was waived because of the decision of the Ethics Committee of Baden Württemberg, Germany. The date of this study is anonymized.

Data Availability Statement: The datasets used and/or analyzed during the present study are available from the corresponding author on reasonable request.

Conflicts of Interest: The authors declare no conflict of interest.

References

1. Smith, T.; Pelpola, K.; Ball, M.; Ong, A.; Myint, P.K. Pre-operative indicators for mortality following hip fracture surgery: A systematic review and meta-analysis. *Age Ageing* **2014**, *43*, 464–471. [CrossRef] [PubMed]
2. Ciatti, C.; Maniscalco, P.; Quattrini, F.; Gattoni, S.; Magro, A.; Capelli, P.; Banchini, F.; Fiazza, C.; Pavone, V.; Puma Pagliarello, C.; et al. The epidemiology of proximal femur fractures during COVID-19 emergency in Italy: A multicentric study. *Acta Biomed.* **2021**, *92*, e2021398. [CrossRef] [PubMed]
3. Royal College of Physicians, National Hip Fracture Database (NHFD) Annual Report 2019. Available online: https://www.rcplondon.ac.uk/projects/outputs/nhfd-annual-report-2019 (accessed on 13 December 2019).
4. Kabelitz, M.; Fritz, Y.; Grueninger, P.; Meier, C.; Fries, P.; Dietrich, M. Cementless Stem for Femoral Neck Fractures in a Patient's 10th Decade of Life: High Rate of Periprosthetic Fractures. *Geriatr. Orthop. Surg. Rehabil.* **2018**, *9*, 2151459318765381. [CrossRef] [PubMed]
5. Li, L.; Zhao, X.; Yang, X.; Yang, L.; Xing, F.; Tang, X. Cemented versus uncemented hemiarthroplasty for the management of femoral neck fractures in the elderly: A meta-analysis and systematic review. *Arch. Orthop. Trauma. Surg.* **2021**, *141*, 1043–1055. [CrossRef] [PubMed]
6. Singh, G.; Deshmukh, R. Uncemented Austin–Moore and cemented Thompson unipolar hemiarthroplasty for displaced fracture neck of femur—Comparison of complications and patient satisfaction. *Injury* **2006**, *37*, 169–174. [CrossRef]
7. Fernandez, M.A.; Achten, J.; Parsons, N.; Griffin, X.L.; Png, M.-E.; Gould, J.; McGibbon, A.; Costa, M.L. Cemented or Uncemented Hemiarthroplasty for Intracapsular Hip Fracture. *N. Engl. J. Med.* **2022**, *386*, 521–530. [CrossRef]
8. Khan, R.J.K.; MacDowell, A.; Crossman, P.; Datta, A.; Jallali, N.; Arch, B.N.; Keene, G.S. Cemented or uncemented hemiarthroplasty for displaced intracapsular femoral neck fractures. *Int. Orthop.* **2002**, *26*, 229–232. [CrossRef]
9. De Jong, L.; Klem, T.M.A.L.; Kuijper, T.M.; Roukema, G.R. Factors affecting the rate of surgical site infection in patients after hemiarthroplasty of the hip following a fracture of the neck of the femur. *Bone Jt. J.* **2017**, *99-B*, 1088–1094. [CrossRef]
10. De Angelis, J.P.; Ademi, A.; Staff, I.; Lewis, C.G. Cemented Versus Uncemented Hemiarthroplasty for Displaced Femoral Neck Fractures. *J. Orthop. Trauma* **2012**, *26*, 135–140. [CrossRef]
11. Taylor, F.; Wright, M.; Zhu, M. Hemiarthroplasty of the Hip with and without Cement: A Randomized Clinical Trial. *J. Bone Jt. Surg.* **2012**, *94*, 577–583. [CrossRef]
12. Donaldson, A.J.; Thomson, H.E.; Harper, N.J.; Kenny, N.W. Bone cement implantation syndrome. *Br. J. Anaesth.* **2009**, *102*, 12–22. [CrossRef] [PubMed]
13. Clark, D.I.; Ahmed, A.B.; Baxendale, B.; Moran, C.G. Cardiac output during hemiarthroplasty of the hip. *J. Bone Jt. Surgery. Br. Vol.* **2001**, *83*, 414–418. [CrossRef]
14. Kotyra, M.; Houltz, E.; Ricksten, S.-E. Pulmonary haemodynamics and right ventricular function during cemented hemiarthroplasty for femoral neck fracture. *Acta Anaesthesiol. Scand.* **2010**, *54*, 1210–1216. [CrossRef]
15. Veldman, H.D.; Heyligers, I.C.; Grimm, B.; Boymans, T.A.E.J. Cemented versus cementless hemiarthroplasty for a displaced fracture of the femoral neck. *Bone Jt. J.* **2017**, *99-B*, 421–431. [CrossRef]
16. Morshed, S.; Bozic, K.J.; Ries, M.D.; Malchau, H.; Colford, J.M. Comparison of cemented and uncemented fixation in total hip replacement. *Acta Orthop.* **2007**, *78*, 315–326. [CrossRef]
17. Kristensen, T.B.; Dybvik, E.; Kristoffersen, M.; Dale, H.; Engesæter, L.B.; Furnes, O.; Gjertsen, J.-E. Cemented or Uncemented Hemiarthroplasty for Femoral Neck Fracture? Data from the Norwegian Hip Fracture Register. *Clin. Orthop. Relat. Res.* **2019**, *478*, 90–100. [CrossRef]
18. Leidinger, W.; Hoffmann, G.; Meierhofer, J.N. Verminderung von schweren kardialen Komplikationen während der Implantation von zementierten Hüfttotalendoprothesen bei Oberschenkelhalsfrakturen. *Der Unf.* **2002**, *105*, 675–679. [CrossRef]
19. Charlson, M.E.; Pompei, P.; Ales, K.L.; MacKenzie, C.R. A new method of classifying prognostic comorbidity in longitudinal studies: Development and validation. *J. Chronic Dis.* **1987**, *40*, 373–383. [CrossRef]
20. Daabiss, M. American Society of Anaesthesiologists physical status classification. *Indian J. Anaesth.* **2011**, *55*, 111–115. [CrossRef]
21. Kannan, A.; Kancherla, R.; McMahon, S.; Hawdon, G.; Soral, A.; Malhotra, R. Arthroplasty options in femoral-neck fracture: Answers from the national registries. *Int. Orthop.* **2011**, *36*, 1–8. [CrossRef]
22. Costa, M.L.; Griffin, X.L.; Pendleton, N.; Pearson, M.; Parsons, N. Does cementing the femoral component increase the risk of peri-operative mortality for patients having replacement surgery for a fracture of the neck of femur? *J. Bone Jt. Surgery. Br. Vol.* **2011**, *93*, 1405–1410. [CrossRef] [PubMed]
23. Weingärtner, K.; Störmann, P.; Schramm, D.; Wutzler, S.; Zacharowski, K.; Marzi, I.; Lustenberger, T. Bone cement implantation syndrome in cemented hip hemiarthroplasty—A persistent risk. *Eur. J. Trauma Emerg. Surg.* **2021**, *48*, 721–729. [CrossRef] [PubMed]
24. Olsen, F.; Segerstad, M.H.A.; Nellgård, B.; Houltz, E.; Ricksten, S.-E. The role of bone cement for the development of intraoperative hypotension and hypoxia and its impact on mortality in hemiarthroplasty for femoral neck fractures. *Acta Orthop.* **2020**, *91*, 293–298. [CrossRef] [PubMed]
25. Olsen, F.; Kotyra, M.; Houltz, E.; Ricksten, S.-E. Bone cement implantation syndrome in cemented hemiarthroplasty for femoral neck fracture: Incidence, risk factors, and effect on outcome. *Br. J. Anaesth.* **2014**, *113*, 800–806. [CrossRef] [PubMed]

26. Ekman, E.; Laaksonen, I.; Isotalo, K.; Liukas, A.; Vahlberg, T.; Mäkelä, K. Cementing does not increase the immediate postoperative risk of death after total hip arthroplasty or hemiarthroplasty: A hospital-based study of 10,677 patients. *Acta Orthop.* **2019**, *90*, 270–274. [CrossRef]
27. Maccagnano, G.; Maruccia, F.; Rauseo, M.; Noia, G.; Coviello, M.; Laneve, A.; Quitadamo, A.P.; Trivellin, G.; Malavolta, M.; Pesce, V. Direct Anterior versus Lateral Approach for Femoral Neck Fracture: Role in COVID-19 Disease. *J. Clin. Med.* **2022**, *11*, 4785. [CrossRef]
28. Breusch, S.; Malchau, H. Optimal Cementing Technique—The Evidence: What Is Modern Cementing Technique? In *The Well-Cemented Total Hip Arthroplasty*; Springer: Berlin/Heidelberg, Germany, 2005; pp. S146–S149.
29. Christie, J.; Burnett, R.; Potts, H.; Pell, A. Echocardiography of transatrial embolism during cemented and uncemented hemiarthroplasty of the hip. *J. Bone Jt. Surgery. Br. Vol.* **1994**, *76-B*, 409–412. [CrossRef]
30. Khanna, G.; Cernovský, J. Bone cement and the implications for anaesthesia. Continuing Education in Anaesthesia. *Crit. Care Pain* **2012**, *12*, 213–216. Available online: https://www.sciencedirect.com/science/article/pii/S1743181617301506 (accessed on 1 August 2012). [CrossRef]
31. Mau, H.; Schelling, K.; Heisel, C.; Wang, J.-S.; Breusch, S. Comparison of various vacuum mixing systems and bone cements as regards reliability, porosity and bending strength. *Acta Orthop. Scand.* **2004**, *75*, 160–172. [CrossRef]
32. Hagio, K.; Sugano, N.; Takashina, M.; Nishii, T.; Yoshikawa, H.; Ochi, T. Embolic events during total hip arthroplasty: An echocardiographic study. *J. Arthroplast.* **2003**, *18*, 186–192. [CrossRef]
33. Parvizi, J.; Holiday, A.D.; Ereth, M.H.; Lewallen, D.G. Sudden Death During Primary Hip Arthroplasty. *Clin. Orthop. Relat. Res.* **1999**, *369*, 39–48. [CrossRef] [PubMed]
34. Parvizi, J.; Ereth, M.H.; Lewallen, D.G. Thirty-Day Mortality Following Hip Arthroplasty for Acute Fracture. *J. Bone Jt. Surg.* **2004**, *86*, 1983–1988. [CrossRef] [PubMed]
35. Byrick, R.J.; Bell, R.S.; Kay, J.C.; Waddell, J.P.; Mullen, J.B. High-volume, high-pressure pulsatile lavage during cemented arthroplasty. *J. Bone Joint. Surg. Am.* **1989**, *71*, 1331–1336. [CrossRef]
36. Herrenbruck, T.; Erickson, E.W.; Damron, T.A.; Heiner, J. Adverse Clinical Events During Cemented Long-Stem Femoral Arthroplasty. *Clin. Orthop. Relat. Res.* **2002**, *395*, 154–163. [CrossRef] [PubMed]
37. White, S.M.; Moppett, I.; Griffiths, R. Outcome by mode of anaesthesia for hip fracture surgery. An observational audit of 65,535 patients in a national dataset. *Anaesthesia* **2014**, *69*, 224–230. [CrossRef] [PubMed]
38. Kumar, N.N.; Kunutsor, S.K.; Fernandez, M.A.; Dominguez, E.; Parsons, N.; Costa, M.L.; Whitehouse, M.R. Effectiveness and safety of cemented and uncemented hemiarthroplasty in the treatment of intracapsular hip fractures. *Bone Jt. J.* **2020**, *102-B*, 1113–1121. [CrossRef]

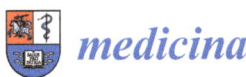

Article

Impact of Anterior Malposition and Bone Cement Augmentation on the Fixation Strength of Cephalic Intramedullary Nail Head Elements

Torsten Pastor [1,2], Ivan Zderic [1], Clemens Schopper [3], Pascal C. Haefeli [2], Philipp Kastner [1,3], Firas Souleiman [1,4], Boyko Gueorguiev [1,*] and Matthias Knobe [2,5,6]

1 AO Research Institute Davos, 7270 Davos, Switzerland
2 Department of Orthopaedic and Trauma Surgery, Lucerne Cantonal Hospital, 6000 Lucerne, Switzerland
3 Department for Orthopaedics and Traumatology, Kepler University Hospital GmbH,
  Johannes Kepler University Linz, 4020 Linz, Austria
4 Department of Orthopaedics, Trauma and Plastic Surgery, University Hospital Leipzig,
  04103 Leipzig, Germany
5 Medical Faculty, University of Zurich, 8091 Zurich, Switzerland
6 Medical Faculty, RWTH Aachen University Hospital, 52074 Aachen, Germany
* Correspondence: boyko.gueorguiev@aofoundation.org; Tel.: +41-78-665-66-74

Citation: Pastor, T.; Zderic, I.; Schopper, C.; Haefeli, P.C.; Kastner, P.; Souleiman, F.; Gueorguiev, B.; Knobe, M. Impact of Anterior Malposition and Bone Cement Augmentation on the Fixation Strength of Cephalic Intramedullary Nail Head Elements. *Medicina* 2022, 58, 1636. https://doi.org/10.3390/medicina58111636

Academic Editor: Minqi Li

Received: 21 September 2022
Accepted: 9 November 2022
Published: 13 November 2022

Publisher's Note: MDPI stays neutral with regard to jurisdictional claims in published maps and institutional affiliations.

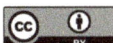

Copyright: © 2022 by the authors. Licensee MDPI, Basel, Switzerland. This article is an open access article distributed under the terms and conditions of the Creative Commons Attribution (CC BY) license (https:// creativecommons.org/licenses/by/ 4.0/).

Abstract: *Background and Objectives*: Intramedullary nailing of trochanteric fractures can be challenging and sometimes the clinical situation does not allow perfect implant positioning. The aim of this study was (1) to compare in human cadaveric femoral heads the biomechanical competence of two recently launched cephalic implants inserted in either an ideal (centre–centre) or less-ideal anterior off-centre position, and (2) to investigate the effect of bone cement augmentation on their fixation strength in the less-ideal position. *Materials and Methods*: Forty-two paired human cadaveric femoral heads were assigned for pairwise implantation using either a TFNA helical blade or a TFNA screw as head element, implanted in either centre–centre or 7 mm anterior off-centre position. Next, seven paired specimens implanted in the off-centre position were augmented with bone cement. As a result, six study groups were created as follows: group 1 with a centre–centre positioned helical blade, paired with group 2 featuring a centre–centre screw, group 3 with an off-centre positioned helical blade, paired with group 4 featuring an off-centre screw, and group 5 with an off-centre positioned augmented helical blade, paired with group 6 featuring an off-centre augmented screw. All specimens were tested until failure under progressively increasing cyclic loading. *Results*: Stiffness was not significantly different among the study groups ($p = 0.388$). Varus deformation was significantly higher in group 4 versus group 6 ($p = 0.026$). Femoral head rotation was significantly higher in group 4 versus group 3 ($p = 0.034$), significantly lower in group 2 versus group 4 ($p = 0.005$), and significantly higher in group 4 versus group 6 ($p = 0.007$). Cycles to clinically relevant failure were 14,919 ± 4763 in group 1, 10,824 ± 5396 in group 2, 10,900 ± 3285 in group 3, 1382 ± 2701 in group 4, 25,811 ± 19,107 in group 5 and 17,817 ± 11,924 in group 6. Significantly higher number of cycles to failure were indicated for group 1 versus group 2 ($p = 0.021$), group 3 versus group 4 ($p = 0.007$), and in group 6 versus group 4 ($p = 0.010$). *Conclusions*: From a biomechanical perspective, proper centre–centre implant positioning in the femoral head is of utmost importance. In cases when this is not achievable in a clinical setting, a helical blade is more forgiving in the less ideal (anterior) malposition when compared to a screw, the latter revealing unacceptable low resistance to femoral head rotation and early failure. Cement augmentation of both off-centre implanted helical blade and screw head elements increases their resistance against failure; however, this effect might be redundant for helical blades and is highly unpredictable for screws.

Keywords: biomechanics; bone cement augmentation; cephalomedullary nailing; helical blade; TFNA

1. Introduction

Trochanteric fractures cause significant socioeconomic costs and represent an increasingly common challenge for both patients and orthopaedic trauma surgeons. Individual surgeons' skills, as well as technical aspects of the implant placement, play a crucial role for their successful fixation [1]. Although numerous advances in implant designing and postoperative treatment methods have been achieved, complication rates between 2% and 16.5% have been reported [2,3] being mostly related to cut-out, varus deformation and rotation of the femoral head fragment [4–8]. In recent years, novel fixation methods were developed to overcome the problematic anchoring of the implant head element (HE) in femoral heads. One of them is implemented with use of the Trochanteric Femoral Nail Advanced System (TFNA, DePuy Synthes, Zuchwil, Switzerland), allowing the choice between a helical blade or a screw HE. Other implants allow a combination of both [9]. Furthermore, bone cement may be injected through the HE into the femoral head to reduce the risk of failure in osteoporotic bone [10–13]. Beside improvements of the implants in recent years, surgeon-related technical aspects during the operation play a crucial role for patients' outcome. The introduction of the tip–apex distance (TAD) and the calcar-related TAD already proved that off-centre positioning of the HE may predict mechanical failure of the implant [14–16]. However, in a clinical situation it is not always possible to achieve a perfect (centre–centre) HE position and surgeons sometimes have to accept an off-centre position of the implant [17]. Recently, a biomechanical study on artificial femoral heads demonstrated the superiority of non-augmented blades versus non-augmented screws in an off-centre position. Furthermore, bone cement augmentation was able to enhance the anchorage of off-centre-positioned HE to a level of centrally placed cephalic implants [18]. However, the resistance to failure of malpositioned non-augmented helical blades and screw head elements, as well as the effect of bone cement injection on a malpositioned implant, have not been investigated in cadaveric bone yet. Therefore, the aims of this study were to investigate in human cadaveric femoral heads (1) the biomechanical competence of two recently launched cephalic implants inserted in either ideal (centre–centre) or less-ideal anterior off-centre positions and (2) to investigate the effect of bone cement augmentation of the cephalic implants on their fixation strength in a less ideal position.

2. Materials and Methods

2.1. Specimens and Study Groups

Forty-two fresh frozen ($-20\ °C$) paired human cadaveric femoral heads from 10 females and 11 males, aged 68.3 years on average (range 54–82 years), were used. All donors gave their informed consent inherent within the donation of the anatomical gift statement during their lifetime (Science Care, Inc., Phoenix, AZ, USA). All specimens underwent high-resolution peripheral quantitative computed tomography (HR-pQCT, Xtreme CT, SCANCO Medical AG, Brüttisellen, Switzerland) to exclude any bone pathologies and calculate volumetric bone mineral density (BMD) within a cylinder of 20 mm diameter and 30 mm length, located in the centre of the femoral head, using a phantom (European Forearm Phantom QRM-BDC/6, QRM GmbH, Möhrendorf, Germany). The specimens were assigned for pairwise implantation using either a TFNA helical blade or a TFNA screw HE. The HEs of each type (helical blade or screw) were implanted in either centre–centre or 7 mm anterior off-centre position. Next, 7 paired specimens implanted with helical blades and screws in the anterior off-centre position were augmented with bone cement (Traumacem V+, DePuy Synthes, Zuchwil, Switzerland). Thus, six study groups were created, consisting of 7 specimens each and combined in 3 clusters, comprising specimens of the same donors in both paired groups of each cluster: group 1 with a centre–centre-positioned helical blade, paired with group 2 featuring a centre–centre screw (cluster 1); group 3 with an off-centre-positioned helical blade, paired with group 4 featuring an off-centre screw (cluster 2); and group 5 with an off-centre-positioned augmented helical blade, paired with group 6 featuring an off-centre augmented screw (cluster 3, Figures 1 and 2). The sample size of 7 specimens per group was considered sufficient for detection of existing significant differences among the corresponding groups, based on previous published work with similar study design, investigating different fixation methods in femoral heads [19–21].

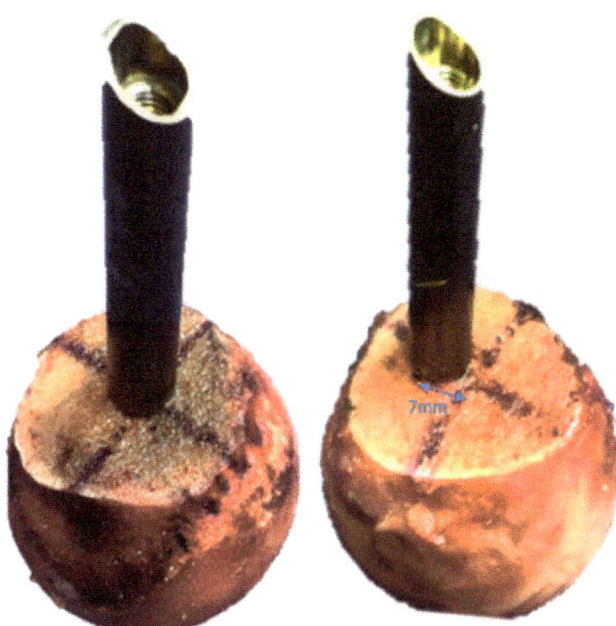

Figure 1. Exemplified specimens representing the implantation in groups 1 and 2 (**left**) and groups 3–6 (**right**). Note the 7 mm anterior off-centre position of the HEs in groups 3–6.

2.2. Specimens Preparation

All femoral heads were sawed 50 mm distally to the articular surface and orthogonally to the femoral neck axis after thawing for 24 h at room temperature. Implantation was performed according to the manufacturer's guidelines under fluoroscopic control (Siemens ARCADIS Varic, Siemens Medical Solutions AG, Erlangen, Germany) with a targeted TAD of 20 mm [14]. According to the group assignment, a guide wire was either placed centrally or with a 7 mm anterior offset at a depth of 40 mm into the femoral head perpendicular to the cut surface, and therefore parallel to the femoral neck axis. For this purpose, the cutting plane of each femoral head was divided into four quadrants defined by distance measurements (Figure 1). For off-centre implant insertion, the entry point was located 7 mm anteriorly to the centre of the femoral head. The 7 mm anterior off-centre position was in agreement with previous work on cephalic implant positioning and seems to reflect well the reality in the surgical theatre [22]. All HEs had a length of 100 mm. The helical blades were inserted over the guide wire to their final depth using hammer blows without predrilling. The screws were implanted after predrilling with a 6 mm drill bit to the desired depth. They were inserted over the guide wire and tightened. Both helical blade and screw HEs were orientated as in a real patient in order to fit within the locking mechanism of the nail. Femoral heads assigned for bone cement augmentation were warmed up to 37 °C in a water bath (Y6, Grant Instruments Cambridge Ltd., Shepreth, UK) prior to bone cement injection. A total volume of 3 mL bone cement was injected into the specimens in a standardized manner under fluoroscopic control. After injection of 1 mL through the HE's perforations on the cranial side, the canula was twisted 180° and another 1 mL was injected through the caudal perforations of the HEs. Next, the cannula was withdrawn 10 mm and the procedure was repeated with injection of 0.5 mL twice [18]. All specimens underwent CT examination to exclude possible undesired bone damages created during implantation.

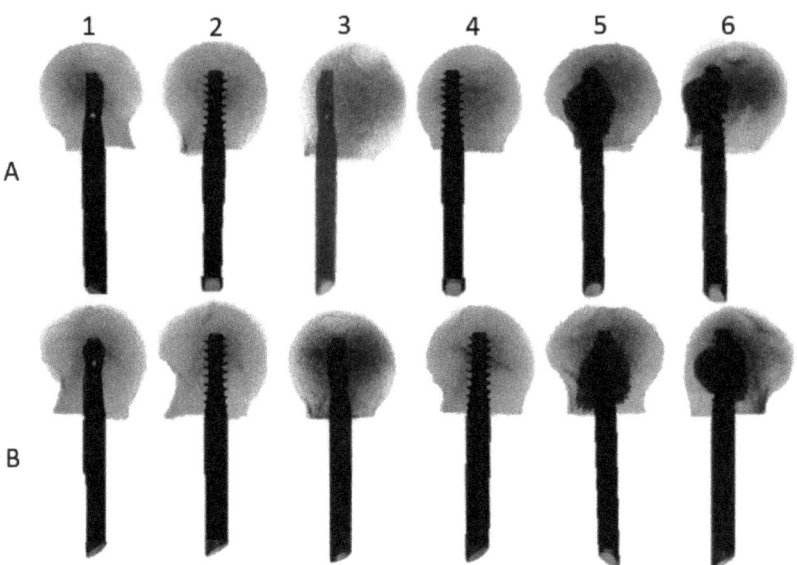

Figure 2. Exemplified samples of each group in superoinferior (**A**) and anteroposterior (**B**) views; groups 1 and 2: helical blade and screw in centre–centre position; groups 3 and 4: helical blade and screw in 7 mm anterior off-centre position; groups 5 and 6: helical blade and screw in 7 mm anterior off-centre position augmented with bone cement.

2.3. Test Setup

Biomechanical testing was performed on a servo-hydraulic test system (Acumen III, MTS Systems Corp., Eden Prairie, MN, USA) equipped with a 3 kN load cell in a dry environment at room temperature (20 °C). The test setup was adopted from previous studies and simulated an unstable trochanteric fracture with lack of medial support and load sharing at the fracture gap (Figure 3) [18,23,24]. To mimic the locking mechanism of the TFNA nail that allows sliding without rotation of the HEs, the implant shafts were inserted in flange sleeves. These were rigidly mounted on a base fixture with a total inclination of 149° to the vertical line to simulate a 130° caput-collum-diaphyseal angle, a 16° resultant joint load vector orientation to the vertical, and 3° lateral inclination of the femoral shaft axis as previously described [24]. The implants were free to slide along their shaft axis with blocked rotation around it during testing. The femoral heads were attached to spikes on a polycarbonate plate mounted on a roller bearing, allowing for rotational movement of the plate and the femoral head around its axis. Furthermore, the specimens were mounted on two cylindrical rollers allowing varus and valgus tilting. Axial load was transmitted to the femoral heads via a polymethylmethacrylate (PMMA) shell mounted on a XY-table to compensate for shear moments during cyclic testing. Furthermore, reflective markers were attached to the femoral head and the HE for optical motion tracking.

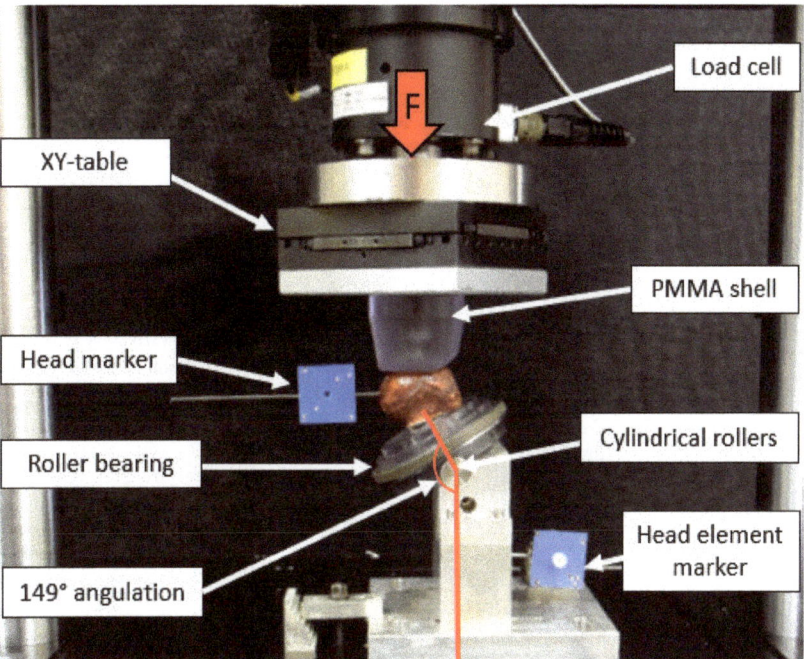

Figure 3. Setup with a specimen mounted in 149° implant shaft inclination to the vertical line for biomechanical testing. Vertical arrow (F) denotes loading direction.

2.4. Loading Protocol

Progressively increasing cyclic axial loading at 2 Hz, starting at 1000 N and being with physiologic profile of each cycle, was applied until failure [25]. The peak load of each cycle increased monotonically by 0.1 N/cycle until reaching 3000 N, while its valley load was kept constant at 100 N. If the specimens reached 3000 N without failure, the test was continued with no further increase of the peak load. Test stop criterium was reaching a 10 mm axial displacement of the machine actuator relative to the test start.

2.5. Data Acquisition and Analysis

Machine data in terms of axial load and axial displacement were recorded from the machine controllers at 128 Hz. Based on these data, initial axial construct stiffness was calculated from the ascending slope of the load–displacement curve between 400 N and 600 N during the first loading cycle. Anteroposterior X-rays were taken every 500 cycles using a triggered C-arm. Furthermore, the coordinates of the optical markers attached to the femoral head and the HE were continuously acquired throughout the tests at 75 Hz by means of stereographic optical measurements using contactless full-field deformation technology (Aramis SRX, GOM GmbH, Braunschweig, Germany) to assess the bone-implant motions in all six degrees of freedom with regard to the marker sets. Anatomical axes (vertical, frontal and sagittal) of the femoral head and the HE axis were defined by proper alignment of the respective marker sets. Varus deformation was defined as the relative bending of the femoral head to the HE axis in the coronal plane. Furthermore, rotation of the femoral head around the HE axis was evaluated. Implant cut-out and implant migration (cut-through) were defined as relative cranial movement of the HE in the femoral head and relative longitudinal HE movement along its axis, respectively. The outcome values of these four parameters were analyzed after 2000 and 4000 cycles, and if applicable after 6000, 8000 and 10,000 cycles in peak loading condition, to evaluate the degradation of the construct stability over the course of cycles [19]. Margins of 5° varus deformation and 10° rotation of the femoral head around the implant axis—considered with respect to the beginning of the cyclic test—were defined as clinically relevant failure criteria derived from previous work [10,23,26]. For each separate specimen, the numbers of cycles until fulfilment of each of these two criteria under peak loading condition were calculated. Based on these, clinical failure was defined as the event when whichever of the two criteria was fulfilled first, and the corresponding number of cycles until that event was considered as cycles to clinical failure. Catastrophic failure modes were evaluated using X-ray imaging and physical inspection of the implant in end of each test.

2.6. Statistical Analysis

Statistical analysis was performed with SPSS software package (IBM SPSS Statistics, V27, IBM, Armonk, NY, USA). Shapiro–Wilk test was conducted to prove normality of data distribution for each separate parameter and group. Explorative data was calculated in terms of mean value and standard deviation (SD). For the single-measure parameters BMD, initial stiffness and cycles to clinical failure, significant differences between the paired groups—belonging to the same cluster—were explored with Paired-Samples t-tests. Furthermore, One-Way Analysis of Variance (ANOVA) was conducted to screen these parameters for significant differences with regard to the other pairs of groups associated with the same implanted HE (blade or screw), but assigned to a different cluster (e.g., all groups featuring TFNA blade implantation were compared amongst each other with regard to centre–centre, off-centre, and augmented off-centre positioning). For the longitudinal multiple-measure parameters cut-out, implant migration, rotation around implant axis and varus deformation at the pre-defined time points of cyclic testing, outcome measures among all groups were screened for significant differences with General Linear Model (GLM) Repeated Measures (RM) tests. Thereby, the number of repeated-measures steps was determined under consideration of the highest rounded number of predefined cycles when none of the specimens within the compared groups had failed yet. If any of the ANOVA or GLM RM tests indicated overall significance, a post hoc test analysis accounting for multiple comparisons was conducted. Significance level was set to 0.05 for all statistical tests.

3. Results

3.1. Morphometrics

Mean age of the donors was 69.4 ± 4.9 years in groups 1 and 2, 74.2 ± 3.5 years in groups 3 and 4, and 66.0 ± 8.6 years in groups 5 and 6, with no significant differences among all groups, $p = 0.121$. BMD (mgHA/cm^3) was 186.5 ± 36.6 in group 1, 180.3 ± 51.8 in group 2, 183.2 ± 37.6 in group 3, 176.6 ± 35.4 in group 4, 180.6 ± 45.3 in group 5 and 179.5 ± 65.9 in group 6, with no significant differences among all groups ($p = 0.999$).

3.2. Initial Stiffness

Initial axial stiffness (N/mm) was 1211.1 ± 85.6 in group 1, 1168.2 ± 260.6 in group 2, 1471.8 ± 553.8 in group 3, 973.7 ± 331.1 in group 4, 1169.6 ± 433.6 in group 5 and 1214.7 ± 309.8 in group 6. No significant differences were detected within each cluster ($p \geq 0.104$) as well as among all groups ($p = 0.388$).

3.3. Varus Deformation, Femoral Head Rotation, Implant Migration and Implant Cut-Out at Predefined Cycles

The outcome measures for these four parameters of interest are summarized in Table 1.

In the centre–centre position and augmented off-centre position, there were no significant differences detected between the two HE designs in the paired groups 1–2 (cluster 1) and 5–6 (cluster 3, $p \geq 0.077$), respectively. However, in the non-augmented off-centre position, the screw HEs in group 4 were associated with significantly higher values compared to the helical blade HEs in the paired group 3 for rotation around the implant axis and cut-out ($p \leq 0.047$), with a trend toward significantly higher values for varus deformation

(p = 0.052), and with non-significantly higher values for implant migration (p = 0.122). Furthermore, the off-centre screw positioning in group 4 was associated with significantly higher values compared to the centre–centre screw positioning in group 2 for rotation around the implant axis and cut-out ($p \leq 0.008$). No significant differences between the corresponding groups with helical blade implantation (groups 3 and 1) were detected ($p \geq 0.579$). On the other hand, whereas the augmentation of off-centre screws in group 6 resulted in significantly lower values compared to group 4 with non-augmented off-centre screws for varus deformation, rotation around implant axis, and cut-out ($p \leq 0.026$), the differences between the corresponding groups 3 and 5 with helical blade implantation were not significant ($p \geq 0.227$).

Table 1. Outcome measures for the investigated longitudinal multi-measure parameters of interest varus deformation, femoral head rotation, implant migration and cut-out, presented separately for each study group at the predefined numbers of cycles in terms of mean and SD. The six groups were combined in three clusters comprising specimens of the same donors each—group 1 (centre–centre positioned blade) paired with group 2 (centre–centre positioned screw), group 3 (off-centre positioned blade) paired with group 4 (off-centre positioned screw), and group 5 (off-centre positioned augmented blade) paired with group 6 (off-centre positioned augmented screw).

Parameter	Cycles	Study Groups					
		Cluster 1		Cluster 2		Cluster 3	
		1 Blade Centre–Centre	2 Screw Centre–Centre	3 Blade Off-Centre	4 Screw Off-Centre	5 Blade Off-Centre Augmented	6 Screw Off-Centre Augmented
Varus deformation [deg]	2000	1.75 ± 0.67	2.17 ± 0.90	1.20 ± 1.02	3.33 ± 2.07	1.06 ± 0.40	1.47 ± 0.51
	4000	2.16 ± 0.82	2.91 ± 1.49	1.61 ± 1.45	5.15 ± 2.58	1.20 ± 0.50	1.74 ± 0.69
	6000	2.53 ± 0.90	3.77 ± 2.07	2.25 ± 1.88	–	1.37 ± 0.65	2.09 ± 1.00
	8000	3.01 ± 1.05	4.89 ± 2.62	3.12 ± 2.37	–	1.51 ± 0.85	–
	10,000	3.44 ± 1.55	6.08 ± 3.07	5.24 ± 6.29	–	1.69 ± 1.05	–
Femoral head rotation [deg]	2000	1.03 ± 1.90	0.84 ± 1.74	0.68 ± 0.42	25.60 ± 17.02	0.54 ± 0.31	1.60 ± 1.67
	4000	1.32 ± 1.93	2.24 ± 5.23	1.35 ± 0.76	30.97 ± 25.50	0.66 ± 0.39	2.92 ± 3.50
	6000	1.65 ± 2.09	3.73 ± 7.71	2.73 ± 1.45	–	0.84 ± 0.51	5.82 ± 7.81
	8000	2.55 ± 3.68	6.20 ± 9.79	5.88 ± 3.42	–	1.22 ± 0.76	–
	10,000	5.03 ± 7.78	8.32 ± 11.44	10.74 ± 10.77	–	2.02 ± 1.55	–
Implant migration [mm]	2000	0.09 ± 0.11	0.16 ± 0.15	0.60 ± 0.02	0.40 ± 0.30	0.06 ± 0.06	0.07 ± 0.02
	4000	0.20 ± 0.31	0.24 ± 0.20	0.10 ± 0.03	0.37 ± 0.39	0.08 ± 0.06	0.09 ± 0.04
	6000	0.31 ± 0.42	0.31 ± 0.25	0.30 ± 0.27	–	0.11 ± 0.07	0.14 ± 0.08
	8000	0.64 ± 0.89	0.48 ± 0.31	0.59 ± 0.42	–	0.19 ± 0.11	–
	10,000	1.42 ± 2.20	0.96 ± 0.67	0.93 ± 0.49	–	0.37 ± 0.29	–
Implant cut-out [mm]	2000	1.09 ± 0.35	1.23 ± 0.23	1.11 ± 0.53	3.53 ± 1.75	1.02 ± 0.19	1.28 ± 0.38
	4000	1.38 ± 0.44	1.55 ± 0.42	1.38 ± 0.75	4.28 ± 2.44	1.18 ± 0.25	1.51 ± 0.49
	6000	1.63 ± 0.53	1.98 ± 0.67	1.70 ± 1.02	–	1.35 ± 0.35	1.76 ± 0.64
	8000	1.90 ± 0.67	2.61 ± 1.07	2.16 ± 1.32	–	1.54 ± 0.43	–
	10,000	2.30 ± 1.12	3.53 ± 2.08	4.33 ± 5.45	–	1.74 ± 0.53	–

3.4. Cycles to Clinical Failure

Cycles to clinical failure (5° varus or 10° rotation of the femoral head, whichever occurred first) were 14,919 ± 4763 in group 1, 10,824 ± 5396 in group 2, 10,900 ± 3285 in group 3, 1382 ± 2701 in group 4, 25,811 ± 19,107 in group 5 and 17,817 ± 11,924 in group 6 (Figure 4). Centre–centre positioning in cluster 1 resulted in significantly higher resistance to failure in group 1 versus group 2 ($p = 0.021$). Moreover, augmented off-centre positioning in cluster 3 resulted in no significant difference between the paired groups with blade and screw implantation ($p = 0.193$). However, non-augmented off-centre HE positioning in cluster 2 was associated with a significantly higher number of cycles to failure in group 3 using helical blades versus group 4 using screws ($p = 0.007$). Finally, augmented off-centre screw positioning in group 6 resulted in significantly higher number of cycles to failure compared to non-augmented screw positioning in group 4 ($p = 0.010$). No further significant differences were detected among all other non-paired groups ($p \geq 0.112$).

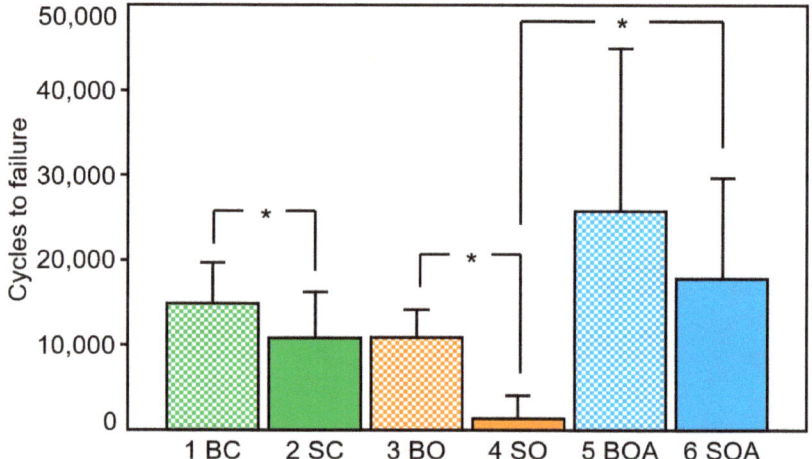

Figure 4. Cycles to clinical failure presented for each separate group in terms of mean and SD. Clusters: 1 (green); 2 (orange); 3 (blue); helical blades: checkerboard pattern; screws: solidly filled. BC: group 1 (helical blade centre–centre); SC: group 2 (screw centre–centre); BO: group 3 (helical blade off-centre); SO: group 4 (screw off-centre); BOA: group 5 (helical blade off-centre augmented); SOA: group 6 (screw off-centre augmented). Stars indicate significant differences.

3.5. Catastrophic Failure Modes

Whereas centre–centre screw positioning resulted in two failure cases by rotation around the implant axis and five failure cases by varus collapse, non-augmented and augmented off-centre screw positioning was associated with exclusive rotational failure around the HE axis. On the other hand, rotational failure in the groups with blade implantation was detected in three specimens with centre–centre positioning, four specimens with non-augmented and four specimens with augmented HE off-centre positioning.

4. Discussion

Trochanteric fractures are a significant burden for health systems as most patients need to be hospitalized and operated [1]. When TFNA is used to treat those fractures, surgeons have the choice to select intraoperatively either a helical blade or a screw as a HE for fixation of the femoral head and neck. Furthermore, it offers the option for bone cement augmentation. The current study investigated the biomechanical characteristics of these two different HEs in the ideal centre–centre and less-ideal anterior off-centre positions. Moreover, the effect of bone cement augmentation on the fixation strength within the femoral head was explored.

Comparable initial construct stiffness independent from the implant positioning or augmentation with bone cement was reported in the current study. Furthermore, similar results were observed in optimally positioned implants, although helical blades demonstrated a slightly better resistance to varus deformation when compared to screws. These findings are in line with other reports in the literature, demonstrating a trend of higher cut-out rates when using screws versus helical blades [10,27]. Furthermore, the current study revealed a significantly higher resistance of uncemented helical blades to rotational forces and moments in the centre–centre position compared to centrally positioned uncemented screws. A possible explanation for this might be the design of the helical blade, which compacts the cancellous bone in the femoral head during insertion [28]. This theoretically provides better fixation strength in low bone quality by preventing bone loss, because pre-drilling along the entire HE length—as required for use of cephalic screws in adequate bone quality—is not always necessary [29]. On the other hand, an increased resistance to the rare complication related to medial cut-through of the HE along its axis, as well as higher pull-out forces, were reported for cephalic screws [30,31]. However, in contrast to other reports in the literature, the current study revealed no significant differences regarding HE migration along its axis among all investigated groups. Furthermore, there are several existing reports in favor of centrally-placed screw HEs compared to helical blades [30,32]. In the current study, the bone compaction around the helical blade might also be an explanation for the higher resistance to rotational moments following anterior malpositioning when compared to screws. Further, the helical blades in the anterior off-centre position were significantly less susceptible for failure and compensated the offset significantly more effective than the screws. This is in line with previous results reported by Sermon et al., who investigated anterior malpositioned implants in osteoporotic foam models [18]. In addition, they investigated malpositioned helical blades and screws with anterior and posterior offset and reported no differences between them. It is therefore hypothesized that although only anteriorly malpositioned implants were investigated in the current study, the results are transferable to the posterior malposition, too. However, despite the higher resistance to failure of the malpositioned helical blades compared to screws, this study fully supports the well-established mantra that correct implant placement in the centre–centre position is of utmost importance.

Various reports in the literature demonstrate an increase in resistance to failure of helical blades and screws augmented with bone cement [10,19,23,33–36]. Furthermore, a recently published review reported fewer reoperations, less complications and shorter hospital stay at the cost of a slightly increased operation time when bone cement was used for augmentation in elderly patients [37]. In contrast, no advantages in resistance to both failure load and axial displacement after cement augmentation of intramedullary nailed trochanteric fractures was reported by Fensky et al. [38]. Moreover, cement augmentation of cannulated screws in a femoral neck fracture model did not demonstrate any improvement in construct stability [39].

However, most of these studies focused on an optimally positioned HE, with only one of them focusing on cement augmentation of a malpositioned implant [18]. The findings of the current study also demonstrate an increased resistance to failure after cement augmentation of both investigated HEs in off-centre position, although this effect was only significant for screws, demonstrating unacceptably low resistance to failure following off-centre screw positioning without cement augmentation in the currently used pool of specimens. In consequence, the findings of the present study suggest that the anterior off-centre position must be avoided for screws in a real patient under all circumstances. If the guide wire of the TFNA system is not revisable in an anterior or posterior malposition, a screw should be avoided, and a blade should be inserted instead. If a screw is already inserted in an off-centre position and is not revisable, the results of the current study suggest its augmentation with bone cement. However, the data scattering in the current study might be an indicator of an unpredictable outcome of this approach in real patients, which should be taken into account by a very careful aftercare of patients with a malpositioned augmented screw. In addition, bone cement augmentation of a non-revisable helical blade in an anterior off-centre position might not always be beneficial. Although in the current investigation their resistance to failure was higher when compared to non-augmented off-centre helical blades, the scattering of the data prohibited significance, and therefore the downsides of bone cement augmentation should be carefully balanced against its possible advantages in a clinical situation.

Another point worth mentioning is that during the biomechanical analysis this study focused on clinically relevant findings. For this reason, no comparisons were made between non-augmented off-centre-positioned screws (group 4) and augmented off-centre-positioned helical blades (group 5), despite the expected significant difference between them (see Figure 4). In a clinical setting, a misplaced screw would be unlikely to be removed and replaced with an augmented off-centre helical blade—due to the necessary predrilling for screw HEs, bone impaction during insertion of the helical blades cannot occur.

This study has some limitations inherent to all biomechanical investigations. First, only a limited number of femoral heads were used per group, restricting the generalization of the study findings; however, an appropriate paired study design was set to compare the biomechanical competence of the two different implants. Moreover, a bone model is not capable to completely simulate in vivo situations with swelling and biological reactions of the surrounding soft tissues following a bone fracture in a real human. Furthermore, the applied biomechanical model did not consider all in vivo forces and moments acting on the femoral head; however, the test setup and loading protocol were defined in such a way to ensure a close simulation of dynamic physiologic loading conditions. Due to the paired study design, only screws and helical blades inserted in the same position could be investigated in the same donor; however, prior to testing, a BMD evaluation demonstrated equally distributed values, thus ensuring comparability among the different groups. Other limitations are artificially created fractures via osteotomies, which do not necessarily obey the physical laws of real fracture mechanisms; however, they were used for standardization purposes and better implant comparability. Despite these limitations, the main failure modes in the current study reflected well clinical failure types in real patients—rotation and varus tilting of the femoral head [40]. However, large scattering of the data was observed in both bone-cement-augmented groups; therefore, further studies are needed to investigate the biomechanical behavior of malpositioned cephalic implants and the influence of different cement distribution models, especially in osteoporotic bone. Moreover, several factors determine the clinical outcome besides the implant design, such as duration of surgery, consequences following cement augmentation, quality of reduction, soft tissue damage, infections, and other postoperative complications. Further prospective randomized clinical trials are needed to relate the findings of the current study to the clinical practice.

5. Conclusions

From a biomechanical perspective, proper centre–centre implant positioning in the femoral head is of utmost importance. In cases when this is not achievable in a clinical setting, a helical blade is more forgiving in the less ideal (anterior) malposition when compared to a screw, the latter revealing unacceptably low resistance to femoral head rotation and early failure. Cement augmentation of both off-centre implanted helical blades and screw head elements increases their resistance against failure; however, this effect might be redundant for helical blades and is highly unpredictable for screws. **Author Contributions:** Conceptualization, T.P., I.Z., P.C.H., B.G. and M.K.; data curation, T.P., I.Z., P.C.H., B.G. and M.K.; formal analysis, I.Z., C.S., P.C.H., P.K. and F.S.; investigation, T.P., C.S. and P.K.; methodology, T.P., I.Z., C.S. and F.S.; study administration, B.G. and M.K.; resources, M.K.; software, I.Z.; supervision, I.Z., B.G. and M.K.; validation, T.P., I.Z., F.S. and B.G.; visualization, T.P.; original draft, T.P.; review and editing, I.Z., P.C.H., B.G. and M.K. All authors have read and agreed to the published version of the manuscript.

Funding: The authors are not compensated and there are no other institutional subsidies, corporate affiliations, or funding sources supporting this work unless clearly documented and disclosed. This study was performed with the assistance of the AO Foundation.

Institutional Review Board Statement: The study was conducted in line with the principles of the Declaration of Helsinki. Approval was granted by the local Ethics Committee (Science Care).

Informed Consent Statement: Informed consent was obtained from all participants in the study.

Data Availability Statement: The datasets used and/or analyzed during the current study are available from the corresponding author on reasonable request.

Acknowledgments: This study was performed with the assistance of the AO Foundation.

Conflicts of Interest: The authors declare no conflict of interest.

References

1. Knobe, M.; Siebert, C.H. [Hip fractures in the elderly: Osteosynthesis versus joint replacement]. *Orthopade* **2014**, *43*, 314–324. [CrossRef]
2. Parker, M.J.; Handoll, H.H. Gamma and other cephalocondylic intramedullary nails versus extramedullary implants for extracapsular hip fractures in adults. *Cochrane Database Syst. Rev.* **2008**. [CrossRef]
3. Szita, J.; Cserhati, P.; Bosch, U.; Manninger, J.; Bodzay, T.; Fekete, K. Intracapsular femoral neck fractures: The importance of early reduction and stable osteosynthesis. *Injury* **2002**, *33*, C41–C46. [CrossRef]
4. Lorich, D.G.; Geller, D.S.; Nielson, J.H. Osteoporotic pertrochanteric hip fractures: Management and current controversies. *Instr. Course Lect.* **2004**, *53*, 441–454. [CrossRef] [PubMed]
5. Hsueh, K.K.; Fang, C.K.; Chen, C.M.; Su, Y.P.; Wu, H.F.; Chiu, F.Y. Risk factors in cutout of sliding hip screw in intertrochanteric fractures: An evaluation of 937 patients. *Int. Orthop.* **2010**, *34*, 1273–1276. [CrossRef] [PubMed]
6. Baumgaertner, M.R.; Solberg, B.D. Awareness of tip-apex distance reduces failure of fixation of trochanteric fractures of the hip. *J. Bone Jt. Surg. Br.* **1997**, *79*, 969–971. [CrossRef]
7. Rupprecht, M.; Grossterlinden, L.; Ruecker, A.H.; de Oliveira, A.N.; Sellenschloh, K.; Nuchtern, J.; Puschel, K.; Morlock, M.; Rueger, J.M.; Lehmann, W. A comparative biomechanical analysis of fixation devices for unstable femoral neck fractures: The Intertan versus cannulated screws or a dynamic hip screw. *J. Trauma* **2011**, *71*, 625–634. [CrossRef]
8. Lenich, A.; Vester, H.; Nerlich, M.; Mayr, E.; Stockle, U.; Fuchtmeier, B. Clinical comparison of the second and third generation of intramedullary devices for trochanteric fractures of the hip–Blade vs screw. *Injury* **2010**, *41*, 1292–1296. [CrossRef]
9. Knobe, M.; Altgassen, S.; Maier, K.J.; Gradl-Dietsch, G.; Kaczmarek, C.; Nebelung, S.; Klos, K.; Kim, B.S.; Gueorguiev, B.; Horst, K.; et al. Screw-blade fixation systems in Pauwels three femoral neck fractures: A biomechanical evaluation. *Int. Orthop.* **2018**, *42*, 409–418. [CrossRef]
10. Sermon, A.; Zderic, I.; Khatchadourian, R.; Scherrer, S.; Knobe, M.; Stoffel, K.; Gueorguiev, B. Bone cement augmentation of femoral nail head elements increases their cut-out resistance in poor bone quality—A biomechanical study. *J. Biomech.* **2021**, *118*, 110301. [CrossRef]
11. Roderer, G.; Scola, A.; Schmolz, W.; Gebhard, F.; Windolf, M.; Hofmann-Fliri, L. Biomechanical in vitro assessment of screw augmentation in locked plating of proximal humerus fractures. *Injury* **2013**, *44*, 1327–1332. [CrossRef]
12. Wahnert, D.; Hofmann-Fliri, L.; Richards, R.G.; Gueorguiev, B.; Raschke, M.J.; Windolf, M. Implant augmentation: Adding bone cement to improve the treatment of osteoporotic distal femur fractures: A biomechanical study using human cadaver bones. *Medicine* **2014**, *93*, e166. [CrossRef] [PubMed]
13. Knobe, M.; Bettag, S.; Kammerlander, C.; Altgassen, S.; Maier, K.J.; Nebelung, S.; Prescher, A.; Horst, K.; Pishnamaz, M.; Herren, C.; et al. Is bone-cement augmentation of screw-anchor fixation systems superior in unstable femoral neck fractures? A biomechanical cadaveric study. *Injury* **2019**, *50*, 292–300. [CrossRef]
14. Baumgaertner, M.R.; Curtin, S.L.; Lindskog, D.M.; Keggi, J.M. The value of the tip-apex distance in predicting failure of fixation of peritrochanteric fractures of the hip. *J. Bone Jt. Surg. Am.* **1995**, *77*, 1058–1064. [CrossRef]
15. Kuzyk, P.R.; Zdero, R.; Shah, S.; Olsen, M.; Waddell, J.P.; Schemitsch, E.H. Femoral head lag screw position for cephalomedullary nails: A biomechanical analysis. *J. Orthop. Trauma* **2012**, *26*, 414–421. [CrossRef] [PubMed]
16. Puthezhath, K.; Jayaprakash, C. Is calcar referenced tip-apex distance a better predicting factor for cutting out in biaxial cephalomedullary nails than tip-apex distance? *J. Orthop. Surg.* **2017**, *25*, 2309499017727920. [CrossRef] [PubMed]
17. Tosounidis, T.H.; Castillo, R.; Kanakaris, N.K.; Giannoudis, P.V. Common complications in hip fracture surgery: Tips/tricks and solutions to avoid them. *Injury* **2015**, *46*, S3–S11. [CrossRef]
18. Sermon, A.; Hofmann-Fliri, L.; Zderic, I.; Agarwal, Y.; Scherrer, S.; Weber, A.; Altmann, M.; Knobe, M.; Windolf, M.; Gueorguiev, B. Impact of Bone Cement Augmentation on the Fixation Strength of TFNA Blades and Screws. *Medicina* **2021**, *57*, 899. [CrossRef] [PubMed]
19. Pastor, T.; Zderic, I.; Gehweiler, D.; Gardner, M.J.; Stoffel, K.; Richards, G.; Knobe, M.; Gueorguiev, B. Biomechanical analysis of recently released cephalomedullary nails for trochanteric femoral fracture fixation in a human cadaveric model. *Arch. Orthop. Trauma Surg.* **2021**, *142*, 3787–3796. [CrossRef]
20. Zderic, I.; Oh, J.K.; Stoffel, K.; Sommer, C.; Helfen, T.; Camino, G.; Richards, G.; Nork, S.E.; Gueorguiev, B. Biomechanical Analysis of the Proximal Femoral Locking Compression Plate: Do Quality of Reduction and Screw Orientation Influence Construct Stability? *J. Orthop. Trauma* **2018**, *32*, 67–74. [CrossRef]

21. Konstantinidis, L.; Papaioannou, C.; Hirschmuller, A.; Pavlidis, T.; Schroeter, S.; Sudkamp, N.P.; Helwig, P. Intramedullary nailing of trochanteric fractures: Central or caudal positioning of the load carrier? A biomechanical comparative study on cadaver bones. *Injury* 2013, *44*, 784–790. [CrossRef] [PubMed]
22. Cleveland, M.; Bosworth, D.M.; Thompson, F.R.; Wilson, H.J., Jr.; Ishizuka, T. A ten-year analysis of intertrochanteric fractures of the femur. *J. Bone Jt. Surg. Am.* 1959, *41*, 1399–1408. [CrossRef]
23. Sermon, A.; Boner, V.; Boger, A.; Schwieger, K.; Boonen, S.; Broos, P.L.; Richards, R.G.; Windolf, M. Potential of polymethylmethacrylate cement-augmented helical proximal femoral nail antirotation blades to improve implant stability—A biomechanical investigation in human cadaveric femoral heads. *J. Trauma Acute Care Surg.* 2012, *72*, E54–E59. [CrossRef] [PubMed]
24. Sommers, M.B.; Roth, C.; Hall, H.; Kam, B.C.; Ehmke, L.W.; Krieg, J.C.; Madey, S.M.; Bottlang, M. A laboratory model to evaluate cutout resistance of implants for pertrochanteric fracture fixation. *J. Orthop. Trauma* 2004, *18*, 361–368. [CrossRef] [PubMed]
25. Bergmann, G.; Deuretzbacher, G.; Heller, M.; Graichen, F.; Rohlmann, A.; Strauss, J.; Duda, G.N. Hip contact forces and gait patterns from routine activities. *J. Biomech.* 2001, *34*, 859–871. [CrossRef]
26. Sermon, A.; Hofmann-Fliri, L.; Richards, R.G.; Flamaing, J.; Windolf, M. Cement augmentation of hip implants in osteoporotic bone: How much cement is needed and where should it go? *J. Orthop. Res.* 2014, *32*, 362–368. [CrossRef]
27. Schopper, C.; Keck, K.; Zderic, I.; Migliorini, F.; Link, B.C.; Beeres, F.J.P.; Babst, R.; Nebelung, S.; Eschbach, D.; Knauf, T.; et al. Screw-blade fixation systems for implant anchorage in the femoral head: Horizontal blade orientation provides superior stability. *Injury* 2021, *52*, 1861–1867. [CrossRef]
28. Goffin, J.M.; Pankaj, P.; Simpson, A.H.; Seil, R.; Gerich, T.G. Does bone compaction around the helical blade of a proximal femoral nail anti-rotation (PFNA) decrease the risk of cut-out?: A subject-specific computational study. *Bone Jt. Res.* 2013, *2*, 79–83. [CrossRef]
29. Windolf, M.; Muths, R.; Braunstein, V.; Gueorguiev, B.; Hanni, M.; Schwieger, K. Quantification of cancellous bone-compaction due to DHS Blade insertion and influence upon cut-out resistance. *Clin. Biomech.* 2009, *24*, 53–58. [CrossRef]
30. Chapman, T.; Zmistowski, B.; Krieg, J.; Stake, S.; Jones, C.M.; Levicoff, E. Helical Blade Versus Screw Fixation in the Treatment of Hip Fractures With Cephalomedullary Devices: Incidence of Failure and Atypical "Medial Cutout". *J. Orthop. Trauma* 2018, *32*, 397–402. [CrossRef]
31. O'Neill, F.; Condon, F.; McGloughlin, T.; Lenehan, B.; Coffey, J.C.; Walsh, M. Dynamic hip screw versus DHS blade: A biomechanical comparison of the fixation achieved by each implant in bone. *J. Bone Jt. Surg. Br.* 2011, *93*, 616–621. [CrossRef] [PubMed]
32. Stern, L.C.; Gorczyca, J.T.; Kates, S.; Ketz, J.; Soles, G.; Humphrey, C.A. Radiographic Review of Helical Blade Versus Lag Screw Fixation for Cephalomedullary Nailing of Low-Energy Peritrochanteric Femur Fractures: There is a Difference in Cutout. *J. Orthop. Trauma* 2017, *31*, 305–310. [CrossRef] [PubMed]
33. Kammerlander, C.; Hem, E.S.; Klopfer, T.; Gebhard, F.; Sermon, A.; Dietrich, M.; Bach, O.; Weil, Y.; Babst, R.; Blauth, M. Cement augmentation of the Proximal Femoral Nail Antirotation (PFNA)—A multicentre randomized controlled trial. *Injury* 2018, *49*, 1436–1444. [CrossRef] [PubMed]
34. Sermon, A.; Boner, V.; Schwieger, K.; Boger, A.; Boonen, S.; Broos, P.; Richards, G.; Windolf, M. Biomechanical evaluation of bone-cement augmented Proximal Femoral Nail Antirotation blades in a polyurethane foam model with low density. *Clin. Biomech.* 2012, *27*, 71–76. [CrossRef] [PubMed]
35. Erhart, J.; Unger, E.; Schefzig, P.; Varga, P.; Trulson, I.; Gormasz, A.; Trulson, A.; Reschl, M.; Hagmann, M.; Vecsei, V.; et al. Rotational Stability of Scaphoid Osteosyntheses: An In Vitro Comparison of Small Fragment Cannulated Screws to Novel Bone Screw Sets. *PLoS ONE* 2016, *11*, e0156080. [CrossRef]
36. Von der Linden, P.; Gisep, A.; Boner, V.; Windolf, M.; Appelt, A.; Suhm, N. Biomechanical evaluation of a new augmentation method for enhanced screw fixation in osteoporotic proximal femoral fractures. *J. Orthop. Res.* 2006, *24*, 2230–2237. [CrossRef]
37. Rompen, I.F.; Knobe, M.; Link, B.C.; Beeres, F.J.P.; Baumgaertner, R.; Diwersi, N.; Migliorini, F.; Nebelung, S.; Babst, R.; van de Wall, B.J.M. Cement augmentation for trochanteric femur fractures: A meta-analysis of randomized clinical trials and observational studies. *PLoS ONE* 2021, *16*, e0251894. [CrossRef]
38. Fensky, F.; Nuchtern, J.V.; Kolb, J.P.; Huber, S.; Rupprecht, M.; Jauch, S.Y.; Sellenschloh, K.; Puschel, K.; Morlock, M.M.; Rueger, J.M.; et al. Cement augmentation of the proximal femoral nail antirotation for the treatment of osteoporotic pertrochanteric fractures—A biomechanical cadaver study. *Injury* 2013, *44*, 802–807. [CrossRef]
39. Hofmann-Fliri, L.; Nicolino, T.I.; Barla, J.; Gueorguiev, B.; Richards, R.G.; Blauth, M.; Windolf, M. Cement augmentation of implants—no general cure in osteoporotic fracture treatment. A biomechanical study on non-displaced femoral neck fractures. *J. Orthop. Res.* 2016, *34*, 314–319. [CrossRef]
40. Brandt, E.; Verdonschot, N.; van Vugt, A.; van Kampen, A. Biomechanical analysis of the percutaneous compression plate and sliding hip screw in intracapsular hip fractures: Experimental assessment using synthetic and cadaver bones. *Injury* 2006, *37*, 979–983. [CrossRef]

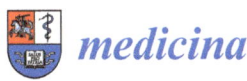

Article

Multipronged Programmatic Strategy for Preventing Secondary Fracture and Facilitating Functional Recovery in Older Patients after Hip Fractures: Our Experience in Taipei Municipal Wanfang Hospital

Yu-Pin Chen [1,2,†], Wei-Chun Chang [1,2,†], Tsai-Wei Wen [3,†], Pei-Chun Chien [1], Shu-Wei Huang [1] and Yi-Jie Kuo [1,2,*]

1. Department of Orthopedics, Wan Fang Hospital, Taipei Medical University, Taipei 116, Taiwan; 99231@w.tmu.edu.tw (Y.-P.C.); 99292@w.tmu.edu.tw (W.-C.C.); 108030@w.tmu.edu.tw (P.-C.C.); 111022@w.tmu.edu.tw (S.-W.H.)
2. Department of Orthopedics, School of Medicine, College of Medicine, Taipei Medical University, Taipei 110, Taiwan
3. Department of Nursing, Wan Fang Hospital, Taipei Medical University, Taipei 116, Taiwan; 93409@w.tmu.edu.tw
* Correspondence: benkuo5@tmu.edu.tw
† These authors contributed equally to this work.

Abstract: *Background and Objectives*: The study assessed the effectiveness of a fracture liaison service (FLS) after 1 year of implementation in improving the outcomes of hip fracture surgery in older adult patients at Taipei Municipal Wanfang Hospital. *Materials and Methods*: The Wanfang hospital's FLS program was implemented using a multipronged programmatic strategy. The aims were to encourage the screening and treatment of osteoporosis and sarcopenia, to take a stratified care approach for patients with a high risk of poor postoperative outcomes, and to offer home visits for the assessment of environmental hazards of falling, and to improve the patient's adherence to osteoporosis treatment. The clinical data of 117 and 110 patients before and after FLS commencement, respectively, were collected from a local hip fracture registry; the data were analyzed to determine the outcomes 1 year after hip fracture surgery in terms of refracture, mortality, and activities of daily living. *Results*: The implementation of our FLS significantly increased the osteoporosis treatment rate after hip fracture surgery from 22.8% to 72.3%, significantly decreased the 1-year refracture rate from 11.8% to 4.9%, non-significantly decreased 1-year mortality from 17.9% to 11.8%, and improved functional outcomes 1 year after hip fracture surgery. *Conclusions*: Implementation of our FLS using the multipronged programmatic strategy effectively improved the outcomes and care quality after hip fracture surgery in the older adult population, offering a successful example as a valuable reference for establishing FLS to improve the outcomes in vulnerable older adults.

Keywords: hip fracture; fracture liaison service; outcomes; stratified care

Citation: Chen, Y.-P.; Chang, W.-C.; Wen, T.-W.; Chien, P.-C.; Huang, S.-W.; Kuo, Y.-J. Multipronged Programmatic Strategy for Preventing Secondary Fracture and Facilitating Functional Recovery in Older Patients after Hip Fractures: Our Experience in Taipei Municipal Wanfang Hospital. *Medicina* 2022, *58*, 875. https://doi.org/10.3390/medicina58070875

Academic Editor: Carsten Schoeneberg

Received: 14 May 2022
Accepted: 28 June 2022
Published: 30 June 2022

Publisher's Note: MDPI stays neutral with regard to jurisdictional claims in published maps and institutional affiliations.

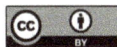

Copyright: © 2022 by the authors. Licensee MDPI, Basel, Switzerland. This article is an open access article distributed under the terms and conditions of the Creative Commons Attribution (CC BY) license (https://creativecommons.org/licenses/by/4.0/).

1. Introduction

Osteoporosis-induced fragility fractures, predominantly in the hip and spine, are a grave health concern in older adult patients. Of all osteoporosis-related fractures, hip fracture is the most debilitating injury and is a growing public health concern in the context of an aging population [1,2]. In Asia, the number of cases of hip fracture is estimated to increase from 1,124,060 in 2018 to 2,563,488 in 2050, contributing to a corresponding increase in the direct cost of hip fracture treatment from USD 9.5 to USD 15 billion [3]. In addition, the prognosis of older adults after hip fractures is poor. The 1-year mortality rate associated with a geriatric hip fracture ranges from 14.0% to 18.1% [4–6], but it can be as high as 36% 1 year after surgery [7]. In our previous study, up to 33.9% of the 281 older adult patients with hip fractures exhibited severe dependence and required additional care at the 1-year follow-up [8]. Moreover, patients with hip fractures were five times more likely to experience a hip refracture within 1 year [9]. Thus, public health measures and a robust treatment protocol for hip fracture are crucial.

To provide improved care for fragility fractures, the International Osteoporosis Foundation (IOF) advocated the Capture the Fracture campaign in 2013 to raise awareness regarding secondary fracture prevention [10]. Fracture liaison services (FLSs) have been recommended as a coordinator-based best practice program for the care of patients with fragility fractures [10]. This involves systematic investigation and risk assessment to reduce the refracture risk and improve survival [11]. For patients with hip fractures, these FLS programs have been demonstrated to be cost-effective [12] and to reduce both secondary fracture incidence and mortality rates [13].

FLS has been implemented in our hospital since July 1, 2019. However, in contrast to the majority of the FLS programs executed worldwide that focus on osteoporosis detection and treatment, we implemented a multipronged programmatic strategy including encouraging postoperative osteoporosis and sarcopenia screening and treatment, taking a stratified care approach for patients with a high risk of poor postoperative outcomes, and offering home visits for the assessment of environmental hazards of falling and assistance. The program also focused on adherence to taking prescribed antiosteoporosis medications (AOMs), and the aim was to reduce the refracture risk in older adult patients with hip fractures. By evaluating the refracture risk, 1-year mortality rates, and changes in 1-year-postoperative activity of daily living (ADL), the present study assessed the effectiveness of our FLS program after its implementation for 1 year in comparison with the results before FLS implementation.

2. Materials and Methods

2.1. Program Description

Taipei Municipal Wanfang Hospital is a medical center in Taipei, Taiwan, performing hip fracture surgery in approximately 180 patients annually. Since 1 December 2017, all older adult patients who were scheduled for hip fracture repair were prospectively followed-up and registered in a local hip fracture registry. The patients were included in the registry if they: were at least 60 years old; had a hip fracture, namely femoral neck fracture (FNF) and peritrochanteric fracture (PTF); and were scheduled for surgery, namely hemiarthroplasty or internal fixation with intramedullary nailing by using in situ cannulated screws or dynamic hip screws. Patients were excluded if they were to undergo hip surgery for a reason other than primary hip fracture, including osteoarthritis, trauma, tumor, infection, and avascular necrosis of the femoral heads. Data on demographic characteristics, pre-fracture ADL, and postoperative outcomes were collected for all patients. All the registered patients were routinely followed-up by telephone to gather data on ADL and postoperative complications, including refracture events and mortality, 1 year after hip fracture surgery. From 1 July 2019, Taipei Municipal Wanfang Hospital began to implement FLS for older adult patients with hip fractures as a physician-led intervention. It involves a multipronged programmatic strategy that investigates and treats osteoporosis, provides shared care by physiotherapists and geriatricians for personalized post-surgery rehabilitation programs and comorbidities management, respectively, and offers a stratified care approach for patients with a high risk of poor postoperative outcomes (Figure 1). This FLS of Wanfang hospital was awarded the Gold Level standard as part of the Capture the Fracture program by the IOF in 2021.

In our FLS program, all patients with hip fractures were encouraged to receive operation within 48 h after admission. After operation, all patients had to complete full workups for osteoporosis by dual-energy X-ray absorptiometry (DXA). In addition, all participants were encouraged to undergo sarcopenia screening during admission where handgrip strength was measured and muscle mass was assessed through DXA. Patients with hip fractures were then classified as those with low or high refracture risk based on the presence of concomitant sarcopenia, comorbidities or their bone mineral density. High-risk patients were defined as having concomitant sarcopenia, T-score ≤ -3.0, or more than three comorbidities. After hip fracture surgery, physiotherapists arranged personalized rehabilitation programs for all patients. However, for high-risk patients, geriatricians were also consulted for comorbidity management, duplicate medication screening, and nutrition support during admission.

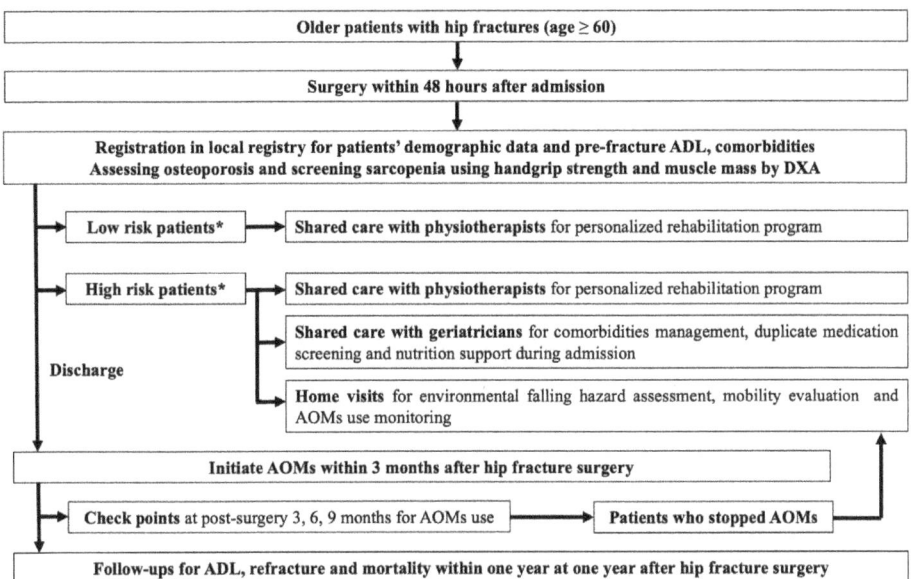

* High risk was defined as patients as having either concomitant sarcopenia, or T-score ≤ −3.0, or more than 3 comorbidities.
Abbreviations: FRAX: fracture risk assessment tool; DXA: dual-energy x-ray absorptiometry; AOM: anti-osteoporosis medication; ADL: activity of daily living

Figure 1. Fracture Liaison Service in Taipei Municipal Wanfang Hospital.

Once the patient was discharged from the hospital, a prescription of AOMs and calcium and vitamin D supplements within 3 months after surgery was encouraged for all patients with a confirmed diagnosis of osteoporosis through DXA. Three, six, and nine months after surgery, all patients with hip fractures were assessed by an FLS coordinating nurse for AOM use. Patients who failed to continue AOMs after hip fracture surgery and those who were classified as the high-risk group were encouraged to receive home visits by our FLS team members (including orthopedic surgeons and nurses) within 1 year after hip fracture surgery, once consent for home visits was obtained from these patients. During the home visits, we screened and educated the patient on environmental fall hazards at their place of residence, assisted patients who had stopped treatment to adhere to prescribed AOMs, and instructed patients on home-based exercise (Figure 2a,b). After the home visits, the visited patients were contacted by telephone 1 month later for follow-up and to record the changes made in the living place to remove the hazards. Patients who stopped osteoporosis treatment before the home visits were also followed-up after the visits to determine whether they returned to the clinic for AOM treatment.

Because the local hip fracture registry had been collecting patients' data since 1 December 2017, whereas our FLS program began after 1 July 2019, patients with hip fractures who were scheduled for surgery at Taipei Municipal Wanfang Hospital were thus divided into two groups: a pre-FLS control group and post-FLS intervention group. This study compared the 1-year outcomes of hip fracture surgery, that is, refracture, mortality, and post-fracture ADL, between the pre-FLS and post-FLS groups by using the data extracted from the local hip fracture registry. The entire protocol for the local hip fracture registry and home visits project for the patients were approved by the Ethics Committee of Taipei Medical University, and ethical approval was registered under the serial numbers TMU-JIRB N201709053 and TMU-JIRB N201912066. More specifically, each participant gave their written informed consent to participate in this study. All participants also consented to the publication of their data.

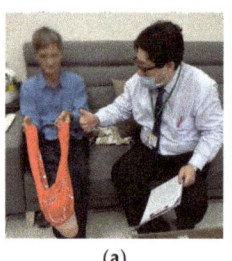 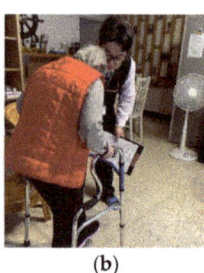 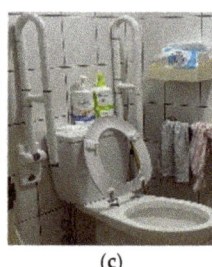 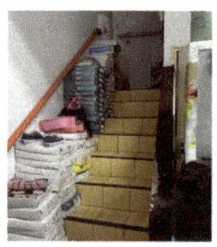 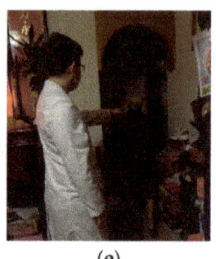

(a) (b) (c) (d) (e)

Figure 2. Home visits for patients with hip fractures. (**a**,**b**) Instructing patients about home-based exercise; (**c**) protective device in the living environment, grab bars in the bathroom; (**d**) hazard in the living environment, obstacles on pathway; (**e**) environmental hazard, inadequate light.

2.2. Data Collection

Data on the following basic characteristics were collected: age; sex; body mass index (BMI); Charlson Comorbidity Index (CCI); fracture type; namely FNF or PTF; surgical method; namely joint replacement or internal fixation; surgical time; and blood loss. In addition, surgical delay from admission and results from preoperative serum tests, including those on hemoglobin, creatinine, sodium, and potassium levels were collected. The primary outcomes for comparison between groups included refracture rates (namely all types of osteoporotic fractures including hip, vertebral, radial, and humeral fractures) and mortality rates at the 1-year follow-up. The secondary outcome was post-fracture ADL after 1 year.

2.3. Key Performance Indicators for FLS

In our FLS program, we defined several patient-level key performance indicators (KPIs) for FLS to guide quality improvement with reference to the guidance from the IOF Capture the Fracture Campaign [14]. Our KPIs were based on the patient receiving (1) osteoporosis assessment with DXA within 12 weeks after surgery; (2) sarcopenia screening; (3) postsurgery physiotherapy consultation; (4) AOM use (indicated by initiation of treatment, prescription within 3 months after surgery, and continuing AOMs for 1 year after fracture surgery); (5) nutritional supplements (specifically, calcium or vitamin D); and (6) home visits. Data regarding the KPI completion rate were also collected and compared between the pre- and post-FLS groups.

2.4. Environmental Evaluation in Home Visits

The environmental evaluations were made by FLS team members by using an environmental checklist during home visits. In our protocol, indoor environmental variables were assessed in two dimensions: (1) environmental fall hazards and (2) environmental protections against falling. Each indoor environmental hazard variable was specifically measured using a dichotomous response ("no" and "yes") to whether (1) inadequate light (Figure 2e) or (2) other tripping hazards (e.g., cluttered pathways, unsecured rugs, and scattered electrical cords) (Figure 2d) were present. Each indoor environmental protective variable was also assessed using a dichotomous response ("no" and "yes") to two items: (1) antislip rubber mats in the bathroom and (2) grab bars on the path and in the bathroom (Figure 2c).

2.5. Definition of Sarcopenia

Sarcopenia was diagnosed if the patient had low muscle mass and low handgrip strength, as recommended by the Asian Working Group for Sarcopenia (AWGS) [15]. The handgrip strength was measured using a Jamar hydraulic dynamometer (Sammons Preston, Bolingbrook, IL, USA). Handgrip strengths of <28 and <18 kg for men and women, respectively, were regarded as low, based on the thresholds recommended by the AWGS [15]. Muscle mass was represented by the appendicular skeletal muscle mass index (ASMI), which was calculated using DXA. Muscle masses of 7 and 5.4 kg/m^2 for men and women, respectively, were regarded as low, based on the thresholds recommended by the AWGS [15].

2.6. Instruments for Functional Outcomes

The Barthel index (BI), for 10 variables with scores ranging from 0 to 100, is an ordinal scale used for measuring ADL performance and mobility [16]. A higher number is associated with a greater likelihood of being able to live at home independently after being discharged from the hospital. According to the proposed guideline, a BI score of <60 indicates "severe to total" dependency. The BI can be used to accurately assess functional recovery in patients who undergo hemiarthroplasty after FNF [17].

2.7. Statistics

All statistical analyses were conducted using IBM SPSS Statistics software version 22 (Armonk, NY, USA). Categorical variables are presented in terms of frequency (percentage) and were compared using the chi-square test and Fisher's exact test. Continuous variables are presented in terms of the mean ± standard deviation and compared using the Wilcoxon two-sample test and Student's *t* test.

3. Results

3.1. Demographic Data

From 1 December 2017 to 30 June 2019 (namely before FLS implementation), data on the basic characteristics of 110 patients undergoing hip fracture repair at Taipei Municipal Wanfang Hospital were collected from the local hip fracture registry; these patients formed the pre-FLS group. Data on the basic characteristics of another 117 patients with hip fractures with complete 1-year follow-up from 1 July 2019 to 30 June 2020 (i.e., after FLS implementation at the Wanfang hospital) were collected; these patients formed the post-FLS group. The basic characteristics of the patients from the pre-FLS and post-FLS groups are presented in Table 1 for comparison. All parameters, including age, sex, BMI, fracture type, CCI, preoperative serum tests, surgical methods, and surgical delay, did not significantly differ between the pre-FLS and post-FLS groups. In addition, no difference in pre-fracture ADL was observed between the patients in the pre-FLS and post-FLS groups.

3.2. KPIs for Quality Control in FLS

Table 2 presents statistics on our specific KPIs for quality control in the pre-FLS and post-FLS groups. Patients in the post-FLS group had a higher KPI (all KPIs) completion rate than those in the pre-FLS group; notably, the post-FLS group exhibited significant improvements in the adherence to post-surgery physiotherapy consultation, use of AOMs, consumption of nutritional supplements, and receiving of home visits. In total, 72.3% of patients in the post-FLS group received AOMs, and the majority (62.3%) of them received denosumab as the treatment drug. One year after having a hip fracture, 53% of patients in the post-FLS group continued AOM treatment, but the AOM treatment rate decreased to 14.5% in the pre-FLS group. In addition, 55.6% and 56.4% of the patients in the post-FLS group received nutritional supplements and home visits within 1 year after hip fracture surgery, respectively.

Table 1. Basic characteristics of patients in the pre-FLS and post-FLS groups.

Variable	Pre-FLS (n = 110)	Post-FLS (n = 117)	p Value
Age	82.98 ± 8.20	80.67 ± 9.76	0.071
Gender			0.66
Female	81 (73.6%)	83 (70.9%)	
Male	27 (26.4%)	34 (29.1%)	
BMI	22.31 ± 3.74	21.58 ± 3.46	0.063
Fracture type			0.349
Femoral neck fracture	66 (60.0%)	62 (53.0%)	
Peritrochanteric fracture	44 (40.0%)	55 (47.0%)	
Lesion side			0.233
Left	52 (47.3%)	65 (55.6%)	
Right	58 (52.7%)	52 (44.4%)	
CCI	5.05 ± 1.74	4.87 ± 1.80	0.475
Preoperative serum tests			
Hemoglobin (g/dL)	12.05 ± 1.78	12.18 ± 1.74	0.924
Creatinine (mg/dL)	1.36 ± 1.70	1.07 ± 0.96	0.477
Sodium (mmol/L)	137.01 ± 3.77	136.62 ± 4.29	0.475
Potassium (mmol/L)	3.94 ± 0.51	3.90 ± 0.46	0.617
Surgical methods			0.173
Joint replacement	48 (43.6%)	40 (34.2%)	
Internal fixation	62 (56.4%)	77 (65.8%)	
Surgical delay from admission			0.982
Within 24 h	66 (60%)	70 (59.8%)	
24–48 h	32 (29.1%)	35 (29.9%)	
>48 h	12 (10.9%)	12 (10.2%)	
Surgical time (h)	71.61 ± 26.23	85.92 ± 54.62	0.073
Surgical blood loss	102.00 ± 91.95	106.39 ± 110.84	0.851
Pre-fracture ADL	82.36 ± 24.23	83.25 ± 23.78	0.959

Table 2. Comparison of KPIs between the pre-FLS and post-FLS groups.

KPIs	Pre-FLS (n = 110)	Post-FLS (n = 117)	p Value
Assessment with DXA within 12 weeks after surgery	92 (83.6%)	102 (90.9%)	0.449
T-score	−3.93 ± 1.10	−3.90 ± 1.12	0.84
Sarcopenia screening			
Handgrip strength (kg)	14.52 ± 7.93	14.42 ± 12.50	0.382
Muscle mass assessment with DXA	80 (72.7%)	96 (82.1%)	0.093
Muscle mass (ASMI, kg/m^2)	5.67 ± 1.04	5.70 ± 1.12	0.84
Diagnosis of sarcopenia	42 (53.2%)	49 (51.3%)	0.873
Post-surgery physiotherapy consultation	32 (29.1%)	117 (100%)	0.000
AOM use			
Initiating treatment with AOMs	32 (22.8%)	74 (72.3%)	0.000
Prescription within 3 months after surgery	24/32 (75%)	67/74 (90.5%)	0.071
Denosumab	10 (31.3%)	46 (62.3%)	
Bisphosphonate	11 (34.3%)	19 (25.7%)	
Selective estrogen-receptor modulators	7 (21.9%)	2 (2.7%)	
Teriparatide	4 (12.5%)	7 (9.5%)	
Continuing AOMs for 1 year after fracture	16 (14.5%)	62 (53.0%)	
Nutrition supplements (i.e., calcium or vitamin D)	16 (14.5%)	65 (55.6%)	0.000
Receiving home visits	0	66 (56.4%)	0.000

3.3. Findings on Home Visits and Changes Thereafter

Table 3 shows a total of 66 patients in the post-FLS group successfully received home visits at a mean of 8.26 months after hip fracture surgery. As for the assessment of indoor environmental hazards, 24.2% and 72.7% of the patients were found to have inadequate light and tripping hazards, respectively, in their place of residence. In addition, only 33.3% and 15.2% of the patients had antislip rubber mats and grab bars, respectively, as environmental protections against falling. However, after home visits by the FL team members, 42.6% of these patients made changes in their environment to prevent falls. Among 30 patients who had stopped AOM use before the home visits, 16 (53.3%) patients successfully returned to a clinic for AOM treatment after the home visits.

Table 3. Findings on home visits and changes thereafter.

Home Visits after Hip Fracture Surgery	n = 66
Mean follow-up time after surgery (months)	8.26 ± 3.40
Mean age	79.86 ± 9.52
Environmental evaluation	
Indoor environmental hazards of falling	54 (81.8%)
Inadequate light	16 (24.2%)
Tripping hazards	48 (72.7%)
Indoor environmental protection against falling	26 (39.4%)
Antislip rubber mats in the bathroom	22 (33.3%)
Grab bars on the path and in the bathroom	10 (15.2%)
Changing environmental hazards after visits	23/54 (42.6%)
Stop AOM use before home visits	30
Return to clinics for AOM treatment after home visits	16/30 (53.3%)

3.4. Primary and Secondary Outcomes

As indicated in Table 4, the 1-year mortality rate after hip fracture surgery was lower in the post-FLS group than in the pre-FLS group (11.8% versus 17.9%) but not significantly so. However, the refracture rate within the first year after surgery was significantly lower in the post-FLS group than in the pre-FLS group (4.9% versus 11.8%, $p = 0.048$). As for the secondary outcome at the 1-year follow-up, patients in the post-FLS group had a significantly higher ADL score (75.61 ± 30.67) than patients in the pre-FLS group ($p = 0.018$).

Table 4. Comparison of 1-year outcomes between the pre-FLS and post-FLS groups.

Outcomes	Pre-FLS (n = 110)	Post-FLS (n = 117)	p Value
Refracture within the first year of surgery	13 (11.8%)	5 (4.9%)	0.048
Mortality within the first year of surgery	17 (17.9%)	12 (11.8%)	0.225
ADL at 1-year follow-up	64.19 ± 34.17	75.61 ± 30.67	0.018

4. Discussion

Before the implementation of our FLS, the AOM treatment rate after hip fracture surgery was only 22.8%. However, after FLS was implemented, efforts were made to promote osteoporosis screening and treatment and home visits were offered to ensure that patients who had stopped AOM use start using it again, leading to an increase in the AOM treatment rate after hip fracture surgery to 72.3%. Moreover, using a stratified care approach for patients with a high risk of poor postoperative outcomes—including provision of shared care through physiotherapists and geriatricians, as well as indoor environmental assessments by home visits—we successfully decreased the refracture rate from 11.8% before FLS to 4.9% after FLS. Furthermore, the 1-year mortality rate effectively decreased from 17.9% in the pre-FLS group to 11.8% in the post-FLS group. Patients in the post-FLS group also presented with higher ADL 1 year after hip fracture surgery than those in the pre-FLS group. This study demonstrated the effectiveness of our FLS program wherein a multipronged programmatic strategy is used for reducing 1-year refracture and mortality rates and facilitating functional outcomes after hip fracture surgery in the older adult population.

Osteoporosis treatment is a key factor affecting hip fracture outcomes in the older adult population. However, missed diagnosis and the undertreatment of osteoporotic fractures following the first osteoporotic fracture is common and now regarded as a critical clinical concern, and greater effort from both healthcare systems and individual clinicians is required [18]. In the Asia-gap study that surveyed women at postmenopause from seven Asian countries, although 70% patients with hip fractures were aware of the osteoporosis risk, only 25% were assessed for bone mineral density and 30% received AOMs as osteoporosis treatment [19]. The FLS program, which is characteristic of multidisciplinary care allowing for systematic coordination between healthcare professionals, is an effective method for improving investigation, detection, and treatment of osteoporosis following index osteoporotic fracture [10]. A recent study on 724 older adult patients with hip fractures in one medical center in Spain reported that the osteoporosis treatment rate can be increased from 12.3% to 74.9% after FLS implementation [20]. In that study, patients treated with AOMs during FLS implementation had a lower mortality rate than those managed without AOMs before FLS implementation (20.2% versus 25.8%), although FLS implementation seemed not to affect the refracture risk between the pre-FLS and post-FLS groups (4.6% and 3.6%, respectively) [20]. Another study analyzing 75 hip fracture patients under FLS with one-year follow-up in one medical center in Thailand reported that the osteoporotic medication treatment rates increased from 40.8% to 80%, resulting in a significant decline on refracture rate from 30% to 0% [21]. However, the one-year mortality rate was not significantly changed (9.2% and 10.7% in pre- and post-FLS groups, respectively) [21]. Meanwhile, in a study in a teaching hospital in Italy, implementation of FLS in 210 geriatric hip fracture patients was reported to increase the osteoporosis treatment rate from 17.2 to 48.5%, successfully reducing the one-year mortality rate from 15.7% to 12.7% [22]. Moreover, evidence from a recent meta-analysis has also shown that the FLS program can significantly improve the osteoporosis treatment rate, resulting in effectively improved outcomes in terms of reducing future fractures as well as morbidity and mortality [11].

In the present study, our FLS program was found to effectively increase the osteoporosis treatment rate after hip fracture surgery, which not only significantly decreased the refracture rate for all osteoporotic fractures but also improved the mortality rate 1 year after hip fracture surgery in the older adult population. Although our results act in concert with the results of previous reports on the effectiveness of FLS [23], we are convinced that the multipronged programmatic strategy aiming at promoting osteoporosis screening and treatment, increasing patient's adherence to AOM through home visits, and using a stratified care approach for patients with a high risk of poor postoperative outcomes has also played a crucial role contributing to the positive outcomes in this study. Regarding refracture risk, good compliance to osteoporosis treatment is necessary for fracture risk reduction, with increasing benefit observed with higher compliance [24]. However, because the older adult patients after hip fractures are at a great risk of losing some degree of motility after surgery [8,25], return to clinics for regular AOM treatment may be a difficult task, which may result in poor compliance to AOM treatment after hip fracture surgery. A multicenter study in a high-level intervention FLS reported that the first-year persistence rates for AOM use was only 66.4% after the initiation of osteoporosis treatment [26]. After FLS implementation, among our 74 patients who received initiating treatment with AOMs, 62 (83.8%) patients continued AOM use until 1 year after hip fracture surgery. The high compliance rate in this study may not only attribute to the treatment choice of long-lasting AOMs (the majority of patients (62.3%) in the post-FLS group received denosumab, which was prescribed for once every 6 months), but also result from the efforts of our home visits to recall the patients who had stopped osteoporosis treatment back to the clinics for AOM prescriptions.

In addition to the high treatment rate and compliance to AOM use, a stratified care approach for patients with a high risk of poor postoperative outcomes is also a critical step in our FLS program. Equipped with the knowledge of prognostic factors, clinicians can adopt a stratified care approach by prioritizing older adult patients with hip fractures who are at a high risk of poor functional outcomes or high mortality for intensive care [27]. Considering the findings of our previous study that patients who have hip fractures with baseline sarcopenia [28], a low T-score [28], and high comorbidity [25] are prone to a poor postoperative function and high mortality after hip fracture surgery, we used these three prognostic factors to classify patients with hip fractures as a high-risk group. A Cochrane review for fall prevention reported that several combination exercises led to an approximately 30% reduction in the incidence of falls and home environment adjustment achieved approximately 20% reduction [29]. Therefore, after hip fracture surgery, high-risk patients were obliged to be concomitantly cared for by physiotherapists and geriatricians through personalized rehabilitation programs, nutrition supports, and professional management of comorbidities. After discharge from the hospital, high-risk patients were also encouraged to receive home visits so that indoor environmental hazards of falling could be identified and necessary home environment adjustments could be suggested. Interestingly, during our home visits, we found up to 72.7% patients had tripping hazards in their living place. Nevertheless, through our efforts, 42.6% patients who had environmental hazards successfully changed their environment to prevent falls. Compared with the 8.3% refracture rate within 1 year after the index hip fracture from a large-scale retrospective cohort study [30], our stratified care approach for high-risk patients reinforced the protections against refracture for patients with hip fractures, thereby effectively reducing the 1-year refracture rate to 4.9% after FLS implementation. Moreover, our multipronged programmatic strategy was also demonstrated to be effective in facilitating functional recovery after hip fracture surgery, which may also be attributable to the reduced refracture rate and personalized rehabilitation programs as well as nutritional support for patients with concomitant sarcopenia.

This study has some limitations. First, our FLS program was initiated from July 2019; therefore, we compared the outcomes of patients before and after FLS implementation based on a retrospective analysis of our local hip fracture registry. However, the comparison between the pre-FLS and post-FLS groups was based on a different historical follow-up period rather than on the outcomes from two intervention arms at the same time period. Owing to the potential improvements in surgical techniques and the quality of patient care with time, superior outcomes in the post-FLS group may also be affected by other potential confounding factors and therefore be biased. However, because all patients' data were extracted from a local registry with high-quality follow-up (the loss follow-up rate for patients 1 year after hip fracture surgery was only 9.5%), our findings likely reflect the efficacy of our FLS program. Second, although rehabilitation programs and nutritional support are essential for patients with hip fractures, especially the high-risk group, the rehabilitation protocol and nutrient regimens cannot be standardized for each patient. Personalized rehabilitation and nutrition support were inevitable and may therefore cause uncontrolled bias. Third, the follow-up period was limited to 1 year, and this may be too short for us to determine the long-term effectiveness of FLS in patients with hip fractures. Finally, the representativeness of our sample was limited by its small size. All participants were recruited from the same institution and might not represent the older adult population undergoing hip fracture surgery throughout Taiwan. Whether our FLS program can be replicated in other institutions to have similar outcomes remains to be clarified. Even with these limitations, we shared our own experience using the multipronged programmatic strategy to improve the care quality after hip fracture surgery in the older adult population, offering a successful example for enhancing and closing the gaps in osteoporosis hip fracture care at Taipei Municipal Wanfang Hospital.

5. Conclusions

Our FLS program, which was designed to encourage the screening and treatment of osteoporosis and sarcopenia, to take a stratified care approach for patients with a high risk of poor postoperative outcomes, and to offer home visits for the assessment of environmental hazards of falling, and to improve the patient's adherence to osteoporosis treatment, was proven to successfully reduced the 1-year refracture rate and facilitated functional recovery after hip fracture surgery in our older adult sample. The experience of our multipronged programmatic strategy for care after hip fracture surgery in the older adult population is anticipated to serve as a valuable reference for establishing FLS to improve the outcomes of vulnerable older adult individuals with hip fractures.

Author Contributions: Study concept and design: Y.-P.C. and Y.-J.K. Acquisition of data: Y.-P.C., W.-C.C., T.-W.W. and P.-C.C. Analysis and interpretation of data: Y.-P.C. and S.-W.H. Drafting of the manuscript: Y.-P.C., W.-C.C. and T.-W.W. Critical revision of the manuscript for important intellectual content: Y.-J.K. All authors have read and agreed to the published version of the manuscript.

Funding: The authors are grateful to Wan Fang Hospital (Grant numbers 109-wf-eva-30 and 111-wf-swf-07) for financially supporting this research.

Institutional Review Board Statement: The study was conducted in accordance with the code of ethics of the World Medical Association (Declaration of Helsinki) and was approved by the Ethics Committee of Taipei Medical University (TMU-JIRB N201709053 approved on 23 October 2017 and TMU-JIRB N201912066 approved on 7 January 2020).

Informed Consent Statement: Informed consent was obtained from all subjects involved in the study.

Data Availability Statement: Due to the sensitive nature of the questions asked in this study, survey respondents were assured that raw data would remain confidential and would not be shared.

Acknowledgments: The authors would like to acknowledge the Laboratory Animal Center at TMU for technical support.

Conflicts of Interest: The authors declare no conflict of interest.

References

1. Lesic, A.; Jarebinski, M.; Pekmezovic, T.; Bumbasirevic, M.; Spasovski, D.; Atkinson, H.D. Epidemiology of Hip Fractures in Belgrade, Serbia Montenegro, 1990–2000. *Arch. Orthop. Trauma Surg.* **2007**, *127*, 179–183. [CrossRef] [PubMed]
2. Melton, L.J., 3rd. Epidemiology of Hip Fractures: Implications of the Exponential Increase with Age. *Bone* **1996**, *18*, S121–S125. [CrossRef]
3. Cheung, C.-L.; Bin Ang, S.; Chadha, M.; Chow, E.S.-L.; Chung, Y.-S.; Hew, F.L.; Jaisamrarn, U.; Ng, H.; Takeuchi, Y.; Wu, C.-H.; et al. An updated hip fracture projection in Asia: The Asian Federation of Osteoporosis Societies study. *Osteoporos. Sarcopenia* **2018**, *4*, 16–21. [CrossRef] [PubMed]
4. Lee, T.-C.; Ho, P.-S.; Lin, H.-T.; Ho, M.-L.; Huang, H.-T.; Chang, J.-K. One Year Readmission Risk and Mortality after Hip Fracture Surgery: A National Population-Based Study in Taiwan. *Aging Dis.* **2017**, *8*, 402–409. [CrossRef] [PubMed]
5. Wang, C.-B.; Lin, C.-F.J.; Liang, W.-M.; Cheng, C.-F.; Chang, Y.-J.; Wu, H.-C.; Wu, T.-N.; Leu, T.-H. Excess mortality after hip fracture among the elderly in Taiwan: A nationwide population-based cohort study. *Bone* **2013**, *56*, 147–153. [CrossRef]
6. Wu, T.; Hu, H.; Lin, S.; Chie, W.-C.; Yang, R.-S.; Liaw, C. Trends in hip fracture rates in Taiwan: A nationwide study from 1996 to 2010. *Osteoporos. Int.* **2016**, *28*, 653–665. [CrossRef]
7. Abrahamsen, B.; van Staa, T.; Ariely, R.; Olson, M.; Cooper, C. Excess mortality following hip fracture: A systematic epidemiological review. *Osteoporos. Int.* **2009**, *20*, 1633–1650. [CrossRef]
8. Chen, Y.-P.; Kuo, Y.-J.; Liu, C.-H.; Chien, P.-C.; Chang, W.-C.; Lin, C.-Y.; Pakpour, A.H. Prognostic factors for 1-year functional outcome, quality of life, care demands, and mortality after surgery in Taiwanese geriatric patients with a hip fracture: A prospective cohort study. *Ther. Adv. Musculoskelet. Dis.* **2021**, *13*, 1759720X211028360. [CrossRef]
9. Lee, S.-H.; Chen, I.; Li, Y.; Chiang, C.F.; Chang, C.; Hsieh, P. Incidence of Second Hip Fractures and Associated Mortality in Taiwan: A Nationwide Population-Based Study of 95,484 Patients During 2006–2010. *Acta Orthop. Traumatol. Turc.* **2016**, *50*, 437–442. [CrossRef]
10. Åkesson, K.; Marsh, D.; Mitchell, P.J.; McLellan, A.R.; Stenmark, J.; Pierroz, D.D.; Kyer, C.; Cooper, C. Capture the Fracture: A Best Practice Framework and global campaign to break the fragility fracture cycle. *Osteoporos. Int.* **2013**, *24*, 2135–2152. [CrossRef]
11. Wu, C.-H.; Tu, S.-T.; Chang, Y.-F.; Chan, D.-C.; Chien, J.-T.; Lin, C.-H.; Singh, S.; Dasari, M.; Chen, J.-F.; Tsai, K.-S. Fracture liaison services improve outcomes of patients with osteoporosis-related fractures: A systematic literature review and meta-analysis. *Bone* **2018**, *111*, 92–100. [CrossRef] [PubMed]

12. Chien, L.-N.; Li, Y.-F.; Yang, R.-S.; Yang, T.-H.; Chen, Y.-H.; Huang, W.-J.; Tsai, H.-Y.; Li, C.-Y.; Chan, D.-C. Real-world cost-effectiveness analysis of the fracture liaison services model of care for hip fracture in Taiwan. *J. Formos. Med. Assoc.* **2021**. [CrossRef] [PubMed]
13. Amphansap, T.; Stitkitti, N.; Arirachakaran, A. The effectiveness of Police General Hospital's fracture liaison service (PGH's FLS) implementation after 5 years: A prospective cohort study. *Osteoporos. Sarcopenia* **2020**, *6*, 199–204. [CrossRef] [PubMed]
14. Javaid, M.K.; Sami, A.; Lems, W.; Mitchell, P.; Thomas, T.; Singer, A.; Speerin, R.; Fujita, M.; Pierroz, D.D.; Akesson, K.; et al. A Patient-Level Key Performance Indicator Set to Measure the Effectiveness of Fracture Liaison Services and Guide Quality Improvement: A Position Paper of the Iof Capture the Fracture Working Group, National Osteoporosis Foundation and Fragility Fracture Network. *Osteoporos. Int.* **2020**, *31*, 1193–1204.
15. Chen, L.K.; Woo, J.; Assantachai, P.; Auyeung, T.W.; Chou, M.Y.; Iijima, K.; Jang, H.C.; Kang, L.; Kim, M.; Kim, S.; et al. Asian Working Group for Sarcopenia: 2019 Consensus Update on Sarcopenia Diagnosis and Treatment. *J. Am. Med. Dir. Assoc.* **2020**, *21*, 300–307.e2. [CrossRef]
16. Mahoney, F.I.; Barthel, D.W. Functional evaluation: The Barthel Index. *Md. State Med. J.* **1965**, *14*, 61–65.
17. Unnanuntana, A.; Jarusriwanna, A.; Nepal, S. Validity and responsiveness of Barthel index for measuring functional recovery after hemiarthroplasty for femoral neck fracture. *Arch. Orthop. Trauma Surg.* **2018**, *138*, 1671–1677. [CrossRef]
18. Bauer, D.C. Osteoporosis Treatment After Hip Fracture: Bad News and Getting Worse. *JAMA Netw. Open* **2018**, *1*, e180844. [CrossRef]
19. Kung, A.W.; Fan, T.; Xu, L.; Xia, W.B.; Park, I.H.; Kim, H.S.; Chan, S.P.; Lee, J.K.; Koh, L.; Soong, Y.K.; et al. Factors influencing diagnosis and treatment of osteoporosis after a fragility fracture among postmenopausal women in Asian countries: A retrospective study. *BMC Women's Health* **2013**, *13*, 7. [CrossRef]
20. González-Quevedo, D.; Bautista-Enrique, D.; Pérez-Del-Río, V.; Bravo-Bardají, M.; García-de-Quevedo, D.; Tamimi, I. Fracture Liaison Service and Mortality in Elderly Hip Fracture Patients: A Prospective Cohort Study. *Osteoporos. Int.* **2020**, *31*, 77–84. [CrossRef]
21. Amphansap, T.; Stitkitti, N.; Dumrongwanich, P. Evaluation of Police General Hospital's Fracture Liaison Service (Pgh's Fls): The First Study of a Fracture Liaison Service in Thailand. *Osteoporos Sarcopenia* **2016**, *2*, 238–243. [CrossRef] [PubMed]
22. Baroni, M.; Zampi, E.; Rinonapoli, G.; Serra, R.; Zengarini, E.; Duranti, G.; Ercolani, S.; Conti, F.; Caraffa, A.; Mecocci, P.; et al. Fracture prevention service to bridge the osteoporosis care gap. *Clin. Interv. Aging* **2015**, *10*, 1035–1042. [CrossRef] [PubMed]
23. Chang, L.-Y.; Tsai, K.-S.; Peng, J.-K.; Chen, C.-H.; Lin, G.-T.; Lin, C.-H.; Tu, S.-T.; Mao, I.-C.; Gau, Y.-L.; Liu, H.-C.; et al. The development of Taiwan Fracture Liaison Service network. *Osteoporos. Sarcopenia* **2018**, *4*, 47–52. [CrossRef] [PubMed]
24. Warriner, A.H.; Curtis, J.R. Adherence to osteoporosis treatments: Room for improvement. *Curr. Opin. Rheumatol.* **2009**, *21*, 356–362. [CrossRef]
25. Chiang, M.-H.; Huang, Y.-Y.; Kuo, Y.-J.; Huang, S.-W.; Jang, Y.-C.; Chu, F.-L.; Chen, Y.-P. Prognostic Factors for Mortality, Activity of Daily Living, and Quality of Life in Taiwanese Older Patients within 1 Year Following Hip Fracture Surgery. *J. Pers. Med.* **2022**, *12*, 102. [CrossRef]
26. Senay, A.; Fernandes, J.C.; Delisle, J.; Morin, S.N.; Perreault, S. Persistence and compliance to osteoporosis therapy in a fracture liaison service: A prospective cohort study. *Arch. Osteoporos.* **2019**, *14*, 87. [CrossRef]
27. Penrod, J.D.; Litke, A.; Hawkes, W.G.; Magaziner, J.; Koval, K.J.; Doucette, J.T.; Silberzweig, S.B.; Siu, A.L. Heterogeneity in Hip Fracture Patients: Age, Functional Status, and Comorbidity. *J. Am. Geriatr. Soc.* **2007**, *55*, 407–413. [CrossRef]
28. Chen, Y.P.; Wong, P.K.; Tsai, M.J.; Chang, W.C.; Hsieh, T.S.; Leu, T.H.; Lin, C.F.J.; Lee, C.H.; Kuo, Y.J.; Lin, C.Y. The High Prevalence of Sarcopenia and Its Associated Outcomes Following Hip Surgery in Taiwanese Geriatric Patients with a Hip Fracture. *J. Formos. Med. Assoc.* **2020**, *119*, 1807–1816. [CrossRef]
29. Gillespie, L.D.; Robertson, M.C.; Gillespie, W.J.; Sherrington, C.; Gates, S.; Clemson, L.M.; Lamb, S.E. Interventions for preventing falls in older people living in the community. *Cochrane Database Syst. Rev.* **2012**, *2021*, CD007146. [CrossRef]
30. Balasubramanian, A.; Zhang, J.; Chen, L.; Wenkert, D.; Daigle, S.G.; Grauer, A.; Curtis, J.R. Risk of Subsequent Fracture after Prior Fracture among Older Women. *Osteoporos. Int.* **2019**, *30*, 79–92. [CrossRef]

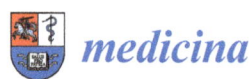

Article

Reduced Awareness for Osteoporosis in Hip Fracture Patients Compared to Elderly Patients Undergoing Elective Hip Replacement

Moritz Kraus [1], Carl Neuerburg [1,*], Nicole Thomasser [1,2], Ulla Cordula Stumpf [1], Matthias Blaschke [3], Werner Plötz [3], Maximilian Michael Saller [1], Wolfgang Böcker [1] and Alexander Martin Keppler [1]

[1] Department of Orthopaedics and Trauma Surgery, Musculoskeletal University Center Munich, Ludwig-Maximilians University Munich, Marchioninistr. 15, 81377 Munich, Germany
[2] Department of Gastroenterology, University Hospital Augsburg, Stenglinstraße 2, 86156 Augsburg, Germany
[3] Hospital Barmherzigen Brüder München, Teaching Hospital Technial University Munich, Romanstraße 93, 80639 Munich, Germany
* Correspondence: carl.neuerburg@med.uni-muenchen.de; Tel.: +49-89-4400-0

Citation: Kraus, M.; Neuerburg, C.; Thomasser, N.; Stumpf, U.C.; Blaschke, M.; Plötz, W.; Saller, M.M.; Böcker, W.; Keppler, A.M. Reduced Awareness for Osteoporosis in Hip Fracture Patients Compared to Elderly Patients Undergoing Elective Hip Replacement. *Medicina* 2022, 58, 1564. https://doi.org/10.3390/medicina58111564

Academic Editor: Carsten Schoeneberg

Received: 13 September 2022
Accepted: 27 October 2022
Published: 31 October 2022

Publisher's Note: MDPI stays neutral with regard to jurisdictional claims in published maps and institutional affiliations.

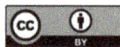

Copyright: © 2022 by the authors. Licensee MDPI, Basel, Switzerland. This article is an open access article distributed under the terms and conditions of the Creative Commons Attribution (CC BY) license (https:// creativecommons.org/licenses/by/ 4.0/).

Abstract: *Background:* Osteoporotic fractures are associated with a loss of quality of life, but only few patients receive an appropriate therapy. Therefore, the present study aims to investigate the awareness of musculoskeletal patients to participate in osteoporosis assessment and to evaluate whether there are significant differences between acute care patients treated for major fractures of the hip compared to elective patients treated for hip joint replacement.; *Methods:* From May 2015 to December 2016 patients who were undergoing surgical treatment for proximal femur fracture or total hip replacement due to osteoarthritis and were at risk for an underlying osteoporosis (female > 60 and male > 70 years) were included in the study and asked to complete a questionnaire assessing the awareness for an underlying osteoporosis. ASA Score, FRAX Score, and demographic information have also been examined. *Results:* In total 268 patients (female = 194 (72.0%)/male = 74 (28%)), mean age 77.7 years (±7.7) undergoing hip surgery were included. Of these, 118 were treated for fracture-related etiology and 150 underwent total hip arthroplasty in an elective care setting. Patients were interviewed about their need for osteoporosis examination during hospitalization. Overall, 76 of 150 patients receiving elective care (50.7%) considered that an examination was necessary, whereas in proximal femur fracture patients the awareness was lower, and the disease osteoporosis was assessed as threatening by significantly fewer newly fractured patients. By comparison, patients undergoing trauma surgery had a considerably greater risk of developing another osteoporotic fracture than patients undergoing elective surgery determined by the FRAX® Score ($p \leq 0.001$).; *Conclusions:* The patients' motivation to endure additional osteoporosis diagnostic testing is notoriously low and needs to be increased. Patients who underwent acute care surgery for a fragility proximal femur fracture, although acutely affected by the potential consequences of underlying osteoporosis, showed lower awareness than the elective comparison population that was also on average 6.1 years younger. Although elective patients were younger and at a lower risk, they seemed to be much more willing to undergo further osteoporosis assessment. In order to better identify and care for patients at risk, interventions such as effective screening, early initiation of osteoporosis therapy in the inpatient setting and a fracture liaison service are important measures.

Keywords: awareness; osteoporosis; proximal femur fracture; hip replacement; fracture liaison service

1. Introduction

The importance of bone quality in the proximal femur is paramount, as it can have a significant hazard for fragility fractures and consequent proper implantation of hip prostheses. The treatment of femoral neck fractures is one of the most frequently performed procedures worldwide. Due to the changing demographics, the number of proximal femur fractures (PFF), one of the most frequent fractures in older people, is predicted to rise to 6.3 million per year by 2050 [1]. Between 2020 and 2040, the number of hip fracture patients who experience a decline in health as measured by DALYs (disability adjusted life years) is expected to double, while socioeconomic expenses are anticipated to rise by 65% [2]. Along with a loss in mobility and daily activities, the mortality rises by up to 20% in the first year [3,4]. Even though osteoporosis following PFF is highly prevalent, the percentage of proper treatment is appallingly low, particularly in Germany [5]. Furthermore, affected patients have very low awareness of the disease osteoporosis [6].

Patient awareness of osteoporosis management is also likely to have a relevant impact on secondary fracture prevention. Considering the known treatment gap in patients with osteoporosis and taking into account the growing awareness of osteoporosis among surgeons, the purpose of this study was to ascertain the willingness of elective and non-elective patients undergoing hip surgery to participate in further investigations and subsequent treatment of osteoporosis.

Patients undergoing hip replacement due to osteoarthritis were used as an elective surgery comparison group (ES) to the patients undergoing non-elective surgery (NES) due to hip fracture. Although patients with a planned total hip arthroplasty often have risk factors for osteoporosis, no regular assessment is performed [7]. This is all the more important because, in addition to the femoral neck, regions such as the distal radius or the spine also have an increased fracture risk in patients suffering osteoporosis. It has been shown that underestimating the prevalence of osteoporosis may increase the perioperative fracture risk. Osteologists and arthroplasty surgeons must be cautious of postoperative alterations in bone density. In fact, it is advised to take into account regular bone mineral density (BMD) screening after knee arthroplasty [8]. It has been shown that occult osteoporosis is present in 25% of patients with hip osteoarthritis and thus osteoporosis screening is quite reasonable in this cohort [9]. In addition to osteoarthritis, osteoporosis patients often have comorbidities with other diseases such as hypertension, diabetes mellitus and depression [10–12]. The COVID-19 pandemic of recent years has also had an impact, particularly on patients with proximal femur fracture. An Italian multicenter study found a decrease in the mean age of patients with proximal femur fracture and a higher incidence of domestic falls than before the pandemic [13].

The purpose of this study was to evaluate differences in fracture risk, demography, and subjective health status among the groups listed in terms of awareness of and risk factors for osteoporosis.

2. Materials and Methods

All patients (female > 60 years or male > 70 years) who received elective total hip arthroplasty or hip fracture surgery in the trauma surgery department of a maximum care university hospital or in an orthopedic clinic in the same city between May 2015 and December 2016 were included in the study. The most significant risk factors for osteoporosis (according to Dachverband für Osteologie e.V. (DVO)) [14] and the patients' general willingness to undergo osteoporosis diagnostics and other screening programs provided by health insurance companies (mammography and coloscopy) were assessed by a questionnaire to determine the patients' awareness of osteoporosis. This questionnaire was already published in a previous paper by our working group [6]. In addition, the 10-year fracture risk for hip fracture and other fragility fractures was determined in all patients using the WHO Fracture Risk Assessment Tool (FRAX®). Patients with the following conditions were disqualified: language barriers, patients with further fractures, and patients with brain organic illnesses (such as dementia, delirium, etc.). The Local Ethics Committee of the University gave its approval to the project. (AZ 351-14).

2.1. Questionnaire

To assess awareness of osteoporosis, readiness for osteoporosis diagnosis, and risk factors according to DVO and FRAX®, the questionnaire was specifically designed. It includes information on age, height, and weight as well as a self-report of current health state using numerical and visual analogue rating scales. This has already been used by our research group to study awareness and risk factors in osteoporosis patients with distal radius fracture [6].

2.2. Self-Assessment of Health Status by Rating Scale

To evaluate a state in relation to a certain trait, rating scales were utilized. Patients can characterize their present state of health using the one-dimensional numerical rating scale in the questionnaire. The WHO defined health as a condition of whole mental, bodily, and social well-being in 1947. Patients were asked to mark a rating scale level on a scale from 0 to 10, where 10 represents major disease (=severely ill) and 0 represents total health. A smiley-based symbolic rating system was employed to make it easier for elderly patients who no longer possess the essential ability to abstract to utilize a numerical rating scale. Additionally, the American Society of Anesthesiologists (ASA) score, which was gathered by associates in the anesthesia department before to surgery, was used to evaluate the patients' physical health status.

Further questions regarding the patient's health status, information, and awareness of osteoporosis were created in a binary nominal scale as "yes/no" responses to help with response and evaluation. As a result, details about osteoporosis that was known or diagnosed, such as current treatment, were elicited. Likewise, participants were questioned regarding their own subjective need for an osteoporosis screening and their perception of the disease's risk. Other preventive exams, including colonoscopies for both men and women within the last ten years, routine prostate exams for men, and mammography screening for women up to 70 years of age were all noted.

According to DVO guideline 2014 [14], risk variables for osteoporosis were gathered in order to ascertain each individual's 10-year risk of fractures and the justification for general and/or targeted medication therapy for osteoporosis. The following characteristics were covered: wrist, vertebral, and femoral fractures that developed after the age of 50, parental hip fractures, nicotine use, glucocorticoid use, and underlying illnesses, such as type 1 diabetes, rheumatoid arthritis, osteogenesis imperfecta, untreated hyperthyroidism, hypergonadism, chronic liver disease, malnutrition, alcohol use (less than one bottle of beer or glass of wine per day), daily dairy intake, and regular vitamin D intake. Menopause before the age of 45 in women, as well as consistent usage of aromatase inhibitors.

2.3. Fracture Risk Assessment Tool (FRAX®)

The Fracture Risk Assessment Tool (FRAX®) is a fracture risk assessment tool published in 2008 by the World Health Organization (WHO) Collaborating Centre for Metabolic Bone Diseases at Sheffield, UK. It provides country-specific algorithms for estimating the individual 10-year probability of hip fracture and other serious osteoporotic fractures of the pelvis, vertebral bodies, distal radius, and proximal humerus. The calculation of fracture probability is based on the factors: age, gender, height, weight, previous fracture, parental hip fracture, smoking status, oral glucocorticoid use, rheumatoid arthritis, secondary osteoporosis, alcohol intake and bone mineral density at the femoral neck. The algorithm queries these risk factors, which, depending on age and BMI, and electively bone density, results in a percentage 10-year fracture risk. This can be determined either in the form of cross-tabulations or using the FRAX-online calculator. The probability obtained in this way can be used to decide on therapy options. Kanis et al. give age-related threshold values for the classification into risk groups, which can be considered as an indication for specific osteoporosis therapy [15].

2.4. Osteoporosis Screening

The assessment of respondents' physical activity, fall risk, dietary practices, and medication use also helped to estimate each person's individual risk for osteoporotic fractures. Our treatment strategy, which is in line with our osteoporosis guidelines, also included basic osteoporosis laboratory tests and spine radiographs as needed to detect common vertebral fractures. [16].

2.5. Statistical Analysis

Subjects were classified into four age groups: Group G1 = 60–69 years, G2 = 70–79, G3 = 80–89, and G4 = 90–99 years. First, the relationship between patients' age and awareness of osteoporosis was determined and analyzed descriptively. Data are presented as mean ± standard deviation (SD). The prevalence of risk factors for osteoporosis was determined bivariate using cross-tabulations and tested for significance with a chi-square test. An unpaired t-test with a significance level of $p \leq 0.05$ was performed to compare the influencing factors. To test for a linear relationship between ordinal scaled variables, a correlation analysis using Spearman-Rho was performed.

Normal distribution and comparability of variance of the data were tested using the Shapiro–Wilk and Levene's test. To compare two interval scaled normally distributed samples with comparable variance, the unpaired students t-test was used. The Mann–Whitney U test and the 2-sample test for equality of proportions with continuity correction were used to examine if the central tendency of two independent samples differed.

In addition, multiple logistic regression was performed using the "glm" function of the "stats" package (version 3.6.2) for the factors influencing outcome awareness, including the parameters age, sex, BMI, ASA score, ethnicity, number of risk factors, and previous fracture.

R software version 4.0.3 was used to conduct statistical analysis (R Foundation for Statistical Computing, Vienna, Austria). The same software's package ggplot2 version 3.3.2 was used to make each graph.

3. Results

In total, 268 patients with an average age of 77.7 years (±7.7), (female = 194 (72%)/ male = 74 (28%)) were included in the study of which 150 patients (56%) were treated electively and 118 patients (44%) were treated non-electively. Patient characteristics including BMI, age group distribution, ASA scores, proportions of risk factors for osteoporosis and patient reported health status as displayed in Table 1.

3.1. Self-Assessment of Health Using a Rating Scale and a Questionnaire

The NES group reported an average score of 4.46 ± 2.42 as their subjective health state at the time of the interview, using a numerical rating scale in which 0 represents perfect health and 10 represents severe disease. For ES patients, a significantly lower mean score of 3.87 ± 2.42 ($p < 0.0001$) was recorded.

Body Mass Index

The mean body mass index (BMI) was 24.05 ± 4.27 kg/m^2 in the NES patients. The patients in the ES group had a significantly higher BMI with an average of 25.12 ± 3.94 kg/m^2 ($p = 0.031$). The prevalence of obesity classes as defined by the World Health Organization among the two groups is shown in Table 1.

3.2. ASA-Score

The ASA score was higher in the NES group, 2.61 ± 0.58 points, compared with an average of 2.05 ± 0.49 points in the ES group. It should be noted here that mean age in the two groups is significantly different ($p = 0.020$). ES patients were 75.0(±6.40) years old, whereas NES patients were on average years old 81.25 (±7.80).

Table 1. Demographic data and characteristics of the study population; Body Mass Index (BMI); Physical Status Classification System (ASA); Dachverband für Osteologie (DVO). * statistically significant $p \leq 0.05$, ** statistically significant $p \leq 0.01$, *** statistically significant $p \leq 0.001$.

Results	Non-Elective Surgery $n = 118$	Elective Surgery $n = 150$	p-Value	Significance Level
Age [years (±SD)]	81.25 (±7.80)	75.0 (±6.40)	<0.001	***
G1 (60–70 years)	10 (8.5%)	31 (20.7%)	0.009	**
G2 (71–79 years)	43 (36.4%)	89 (59.3%)	<0.001	***
G3 (80–90 years)	62 (41%)	30 (20.0%)	<0.001	***
G4 (91–100 years)	13 (11%)	0 (0.0%)	—	—
Gender				
male	25 (21%)	49 (33%)	0.037	*
female	93 (79%)	101 (67%)	0.037	*
BMI [kg/m^2 (±SD)]	24.05 (±4.27)	25.12 (±3.94)	0.031	*
<20 kg/m^2	10 (8.5%)	6 (4.0%)	0.016	*
20–24.9 kg/m^2	66 (55.9%)	65 (43.3%)	0.054	ns
25–29.9 kg/m^2	30 (25.4%)	66 (44.0%)	0.002	**
30–34.9 kg/m^2	10 (8.5%)	11 (7.33)	0.907	ns
≥35 kg/m^2	2 (1.7%)	2 (1.33)	1.000	ns
ASA Score [Score; (±SD)]	2.61 (±0.58)	2.05 (±0.49)	<0.001	***
1	2 (1.7%)	13 (8.7%)	0.028	*
2	45 (38.1%)	117 (71.0%)	<0.001	***
3	67 (56.8%)	19 (12.7)	<0.001	***
4	4 (3.4%)	1 (0.7%)	0.237	ns
Risk Factors (DVO) [n; (%)]				
Parental hip fracture	37 (31.0%)	27 (18.0%)	0.016	*
Current smoker	12 (10.0%)	10 (7.0%)	0.416	ns
Glucocorticoid use	16 (14.0%)	20 (13.0%)	1.000	ns
Rheumatoid arthritis	6 (5.0%)	8 (5.0%)	1.000	ns
Menopause < 45 year	31 (26.3%)	44 (29.3%)	0.676	ns
Aromatase inhibitor use	9 (8.0%)	1 (1.0%)	0.007	**
Alcohol (>1 bottle of beer a day)	16 (14.0%)	21 (14.0%)	0.701	ns
No regular consumption of dairy products	35 (30.0%)	24 (16.0%)	0.011	*
Cumulative number of risk factors per patient	1.86 (±1.45)	1.25 (±1.12)	<0.001	***
Osteoporosis Therapy Information [n; (%)]				
Regular vitamin D intake	25 (21.0%)	60 (40.0%)	0.002	**
Known osteoporosis diagnosis	29 (25.0%)	41 (27.0%)	0.711	ns
Osteoporosis medication intake	27 (23.0%)	37 (25.0%)	0.845	ns
Patient Reported Health Status (1–10)	4.46 (±2.42)	3.87 (±2.42)	0.048	*

3.3. Risk Factors and FRAX

On average, patients in the NES group had slightly more risk factors (1.86 ± 1.45) based on the DVO guidelines than the ES group (1.25 ± 1.12). The prevalence of the queried risk factors for osteoporosis is shown in Table 1. According to FRAX®-Score, "high risk" is defined as having a 10-year fracture hazard of ≥3% for hip and/or ≥20% for other major osteoporotic fractures, while "low risk" refers to risk percentages that are lower than these cutoff points. Of the investigated NES patients, 35% (41/118) had a 20% chance of suffering a severe osteoporotic fracture in the following ten years. In contrast, the proportion in the ES group was only 25% (38/150). The proportion at high risk of hip fracture within the next 10 years was significantly lower in the ES group at 70% (105/150) than in the NES group at 92% (108/118), ($p \leq 0.0001$).

Only 46.6% (55/118) of NES patients and 50.7% (75/150) ES patients considered further diagnostics regarding osteoporosis necessary. This was significantly lower than the proportion of patients who underwent a precautionary colonoscopy (NES: 62% vs. ES: 66%), or regularly underwent general preventive examinations by the health insurers (NES: 67% vs. ES: 85%).

When the raw FRAX scores are compared, the NES group showed a significantly higher average fracture risk of 28.1 ± 16.3% compared with 14.6 ± 9.7% in the ES cohort (Figure 1A).

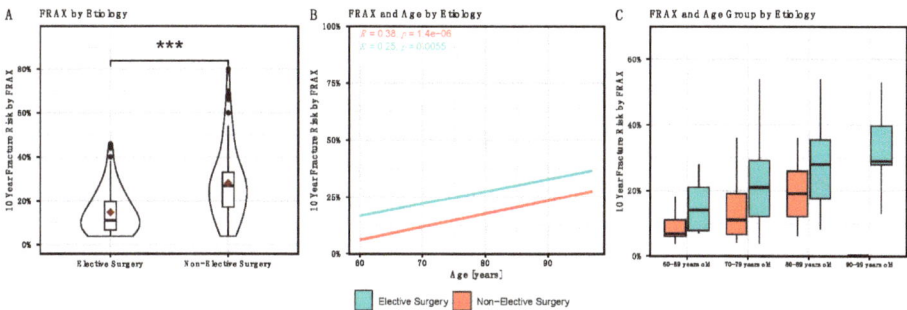

Figure 1. (**A**): FRAX® Score by Aetiology: (**A**): Distribution of FRAX-Score by Aetiology. FRAX score was found to be significantly higher in the trauma related group (NES) than in the Elective Care group, indicating that the fracture patients had a significantly higher risk of subsequent fracture than the Elective Care patients. (**B**): FRAX® Score and age by Aetiology. The FRAX score and thus the fracture risk increases continuously with age in both groups. (**C**): FRAX® Score by Age Groups and Aetiology: A comparison of the age groups also shows a higher fracture risk in the trauma group. (***)-p-value < 0.001.

When the FRAX score is related to the age of the patients, a linear regression analysis shows that in both groups the fracture risk after FRAX increases significantly with increasing age ($p \leq 0.01$). The coefficient of determination was $R^2 = 0.38$ for the NES group and $R^2 = 0.25$ for the elective patients (Figure 1B).

The divisions into the four age groups selected as described above also clearly showed increasing fracture risk with old age (Figure 1C).

3.4. Osteoporosis Therapy Information

In the preventive measures we investigated to avoid osteoporosis, the two groups differed significantly in their regular intake of vitamin D. The difference between the two groups was not significant. (NES: 21% and ES: 40%, $p < 0.001$). The proportion of patients with known osteoporosis and specific therapy was almost the same in both groups (Table 1).

3.5. Threadiness

80% of elective care patients considered osteoporosis to be a threatening disease for them, whereas the proportion in the NES was significantly smaller at 53.4% ($p \leq 0.0001$).

3.6. Patients' Osteoporosis Awareness

In accordance with the questionnaire, elective patients had a greater awareness rate of 50.7% compared to individuals who had fractures at 42% (Figure 2B).

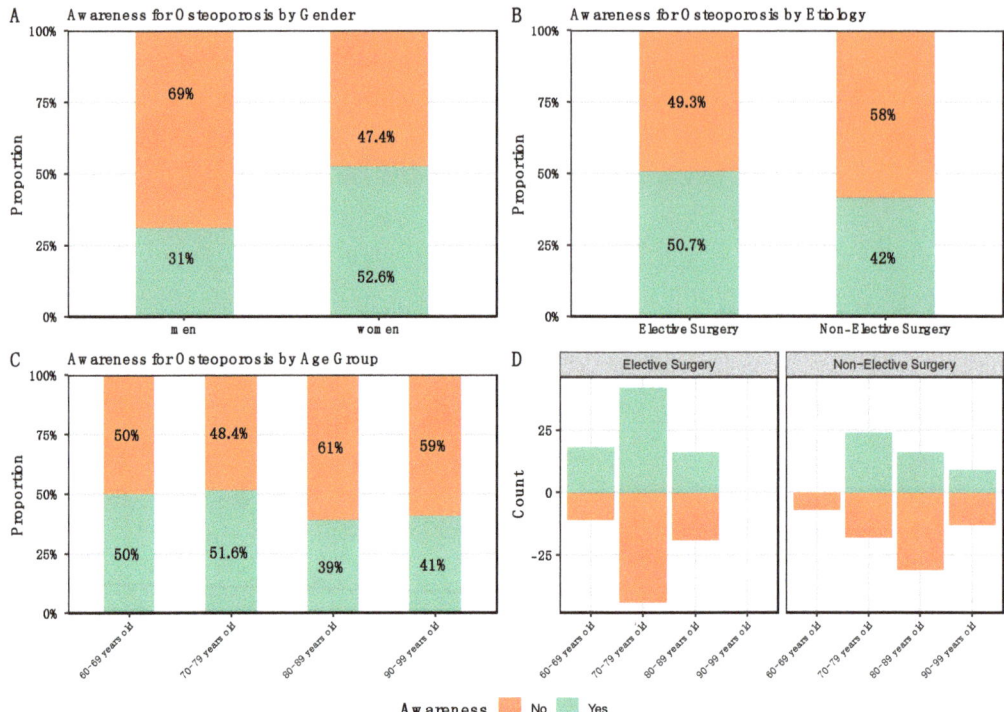

Figure 2. (**A**): Patient's awareness: (**A**): Patients' percentage of awareness of osteoporosis by gender, shows an alarming lower awareness among men; (**B**): Patients' awareness for osteoporosis divided by electivity in percent, among patients not affected by a fracture, a higher percentage has awareness; (**C**): Percentages of patients' awareness of osteoporosis by age groups; Awareness is highest in the age group 60–69 years and lowest in the age group 80–89 years; (**D**): Patients' awareness for osteoporosis divided by Electivity and age groups in percent. Only in the 70–79 age group is awareness higher among trauma patients than among elective patients. In the age group 90+ no elective patients could be included.

Regarding the gender of the patients, it was found that the awareness was significantly higher in women with 52.6% (102/194) than in men with 31.0% (23/74) ($p \leq 0.01$) (Figure 2A).

It was discovered that awareness of osteoporosis (AO) was highest in those aged 70 to 79, with 51.6%, and lowest in those aged 90 to 99, with 41.0% (Figure 2C).

When the patients are divided into age groups and electivity, it can be seen that in the 60–69 years age group, the ES had 62.0% ($n = 29$) awareness, whereas in the NES group, none of the patients were aware 0% ($n = 7$). In the 70–79 age group, NES patients showed slightly higher awareness (57.0%; $n = 42$) than the ES group (48.8%; $n = 86$). In contrast, in the 80–89 age group, the awareness of ES patients was considerably higher (45.7%; $n = 45$) than that of NES patients (34.0%; $n = 47$).

In the 90+ age group, only patients in the NES group could be included, as elective hip replacement is generally no longer performed in this cohort due to high surgical risk. In the NES group, the proportion of patients with awareness was 41.0% ($n = 22$) (Figure 2D).

The multiple linear regression performed to determine the factors influencing the presence of awareness showed that age, BMI, ASA score, and number of risk factors had no significant influence (Supplementary Table S1). In contrast, patients with female gender had an odds ratio of 1.94 (95% CI: 1.06, −3.64) for the presence of awareness ($p = 0.035$).

Patients with no history of fracture had an odds ratio of 0.47 (95% CI: 0.23–0.94) versus those with a positive history of fracture ($p = 0.033$). The ethnology "non-elective" showed a barely non-significant difference with a p-value of 0.059 and an odds ratio of 0.54 (95% CI: 0.28–1.02) compared to elective patients.

4. Discussion

Our study's findings demonstrated that patients having elective hip surgery were much more aware of osteoporosis and more likely to receive the right treatment than patients having surgery for an osteoporotic proximal femur fracture.

Awareness of underlying osteoporosis in older trauma patients has a relevant influence on compliance for further diagnosis and treatment [17]. It is evident that the documented reduction in fracture risk of up to 70% cannot be realized in patients, that are not treatment-adherent, because the compliance of oral bisphosphonates is as low as 50% one year after start of therapy. [18,19]. Even if there was an existing fragility fracture or a known risk for further fractures, patients' willingness to participate in other screening programs (colonoscopy and check-ups) was higher in both groups of patients than in those screening programs for osteoporosis. This reduced awareness is one factor that may help to explain why therapy for osteoporosis is so low in elective and non-elective patients [7]. To frame the results, it is important to keep in mind that in Germany the costs for screening programs for mammography and colonoscopy are covered by the public health insurance. This is currently not the case for osteoporosis screening, which is a major factor for a reduced utilization of osteoporosis screening measures in the general population. In our studies, the costs for the screening examinations were covered by the treating clinics, which meant that the patients did not incur any direct costs for participating in the examinations and thus the cost factor is unlikely to have had any influence on the willingness to participate.

For the best possible surgical management, it is essential to know about the existence of osteoporosis or osteopenia. This is because the stability of the bone already plays an important role in the selection of the prosthesis and its application. Patients undergoing hip arthroplasty today are the patients who are at risk of suffering periprosthetic femur fracture in the future. Therefore, the knowledge of bone health is crucial for selecting a suitable drug therapy that positively influences implant osseointegration and reduces the risk of periprosthetic fracture [20,21].

The fracture risk determined by means of FRAX is clearly correlated with age in our patients, since on the one hand age is included in the score and on the other hand with increasing age basically more comorbidities are to be expected, which are also recorded in the score Given that a fracture in the past is considered a risk factor in the FRAX score, it makes sense that individuals who have recently undergone trauma have a higher fracture risk. However, this increased risk in the NES group is not associated with increased awareness compared to elective patients. The reason for this is multifactorial. First, it has been shown that fracture patients are generally less aware of preventive examinations (NES: 67%; ES: 85%), suggesting reduced health awareness in this group. Second, the fracture patients presumably have fewer physician contacts due to musculoskeletal problems than patients who receive a hip prosthesis due to chronic arthritic disease of the corresponding joint. Due to this mostly long-standing disease, the physicians have more opportunities to create a higher awareness of the disease with regard to the musculoskeletal system during the treatments than with the fracture patients who are acutely admitted to the clinic. Furthermore, elective patients rate their health status during hospitalization significantly lower than non-elective patients, indicating a higher level of suffering among elective patients than among acute patients, which makes them more likely to feel threatened by illness than the supposedly healthier fracture patients. The ASA score collected anesthesiologists, contradicts the subjective assessment of the patients, as it rates the fracture patients as more severely affected than the elective patients. Another relevant factor is the fact that the patients who were acutely hospitalized after a fall consider chronic diseases to be less threatening than patients who are already chronically ill with arthrosis. In addition, on the surgical side, the focus is on the best possible treatment of the acute injury and less on the detection of any additional osteoporosis that may be present. This can lead to a communication and perception problem in fracture patients, as they attribute their suffering to the acute trauma and are not aware of the risk of a further fragility fracture. Patients frequently may not understand the order of causation, believing that the damage was first caused by diminished bone stability rather than the actual fall. Accordingly, physicians should focus on creating the best possible understanding of the disease and the best possible awareness among patients. This is a cornerstone for an early start of therapy, good therapy compliance and adherence, which is essential for successful subsequent fracture prophylaxis. This is particularly important for secondary prevention in fracture patients, but also relevant for primary prevention in elective patients. Mortality after PFF has remained almost the same over the last 30 years, still significantly increased in the first year, up to 21–24% depending on the literature [22].

Therefore, Lyles et al. were able to demonstrate another important argument for the postoperative implementation of specific therapy for osteoporosis after PFF: iv administration of 5 mg zoledronic acid within 90 days postoperatively significantly reduced mortality by 28% in this group [23].

Another important point for primary as well as secondary prevention is a regular intake of vitamin D. Among the elective patients before surgery, twice as much vitamin D was substituted as among the NES patients. The reasons for this could be a possibly increased health awareness among the ES patients combined with a higher awareness of osteoporosis among them. Presumably, ES patients generally pay more attention to a healthy lifestyle and are therefore more likely to take vitamin D regularly as a preventive measure.

Similar to this, after coronary stent placement, chronic medication and close monitoring are much more frequently used in internal medicine to manage disorders, such as hypertension and hypercholesterolemia, which cause artery narrowing and calcification. Additionally, the health care system's diverse systems frequently make consistent therapy challenging. Models such as the Fracture Liaison Service have been developed to monitor patients over the long term, including via many healthcare system sectors, to help with this [24–26].

It is important to take into account the study's limitations, such as the fact that it was limited to one university hospital and one affiliated hospital. A multicenter research would be really intriguing to perform. Although patients with cognitive impairment were not included in the study, it is feasible that patients' understanding of the underlying osteoporosis may differ depending on their degree of education, even though this study did not assess educational level.

To our knowledge, the current study is the first to investigate whether patients undergoing elective and nonelective hip surgery are aware of the underlying osteoporosis.

5. Conclusions

We demonstrated that in all groups, willingness to participate in other screening programs (preventive examinations and colonoscopy) was significantly higher than willingness to participate in further osteoporosis diagnostics. Therefore, implementation of a screening and care program for osteoporosis such as Fracture Liaison Services (FLS) may improve patient awareness of this condition especially among fracture patients.

Supplementary Materials: The following are available online at https://www.mdpi.com/article/10.3390/medicina58111564/s1, Table S1: Results of multiple linear regression performed to determine the factors influencing the presence of awareness for osteoporosis.

Author Contributions: Study concept and design: A.M.K., U.C.S., M.B. and C.N. Data acquisition: N.T., M.B. and U.C.S. Data analysis: A.M.K., M.K. and M.M.S. Data interpretation: A.M.K., M.K., M.M.S. and C.N. Drafting the manuscript: A.M.K., M.K. and U.C.S. Manuscript revision for important intellectual content: W.B., M.M.S., C.N., A.M.K., M.K. and U.C.S. Supervision, C.N., W.B. and W.P. Project administration, C.N., W.B., A.M.K. and M.K. All authors have read and agreed to the published version of the manuscript.

Funding: This research received no external funding.

Institutional Review Board Statement: The Institutional Review Board of the LMU Munich Medical Faculty gave its approval to the study after it was carried out in accordance with the Declaration of Helsinki's principles. The university's ethics committee gave the study their seal of approval, and it was filed as AZ 351-14.

Informed Consent Statement: The patients gave their written informed consent in order for this paper to be published.

Data Availability Statement: The corresponding author can provide the data described in this study upon request. Due to laws governing data protection and privacy, the data are not accessible to the general public.

Conflicts of Interest: The authors declare no conflict of interests.

References

1. Kanis, J.A.; Odén, A.; McCloskey, E.V.; Johansson, H.; Wahl, D.A.; Cooper, C. A Systematic Review of Hip Fracture Incidence and Probability of Fracture Worldwide. *Osteoporos. Int.* **2012**, *23*, 2239–2256. [CrossRef] [PubMed]
2. Hagen, G.; Magnussen, J.; Tell, G.; Omsland, T. Estimating the Future Burden of Hip Fractures in Norway. A NOREPOS Study. *Bone* **2020**, *131*, 115156. [CrossRef] [PubMed]
3. Downey, C.; Kelly, M.; Quinlan, J.F. Changing Trends in the Mortality Rate at 1-Year Post Hip Fracture—A Systematic Review. *World J. Orthop.* **2019**, *10*, 166–175. [CrossRef]
4. Dyer, S.M.; Crotty, M.; Fairhall, N.; Magaziner, J.; Beaupre, L.A.; Cameron, I.D.; Sherrington, C. A Critical Review of the Long-Term Disability Outcomes Following Hip Fracture. *BMC Geriatr.* **2016**, *16*, 158. [CrossRef]
5. Desai, R.J.; Mahesri, M.; Abdia, Y.; Barberio, J.; Tong, A.; Zhang, D.; Mavros, P.; Kim, S.C.; Franklin, J.M. Association of Osteoporosis Medication Use After Hip Fracture With Prevention of Subsequent Nonvertebral Fractures: An Instrumental Variable Analysis. *JAMA Netw. Open* **2018**, *1*, e180826. [CrossRef] [PubMed]
6. Keppler, A.M.; Kraus, M.; Blaschke, M.; Thomasser, N.; Kammerlander, C.; Böcker, W.; Neuerburg, C.; Stumpf, U.C. Reduced Awareness for Osteoporosis in Distal Radius Fracture Patients Compared to Patients with Proximal Femur Fractures. *J. Clin. Med.* **2021**, *10*, 848. [CrossRef]
7. Bernatz, J.T.; Brooks, A.E.; Squire, M.W.; Illgen, R.I.; Binkley, N.C.; Anderson, P.A. Osteoporosis Is Common and Undertreated Prior to Total Joint Arthroplasty. *J. Arthroplast.* **2019**, *34*, 1347–1353. [CrossRef]
8. Bernatz, J.T.; Krueger, D.C.; Squire, M.W.; Illgen, R.L.; Binkley, N.C.; Anderson, P.A. Unrecognized Osteoporosis Is Common in Patients With a Well-Functioning Total Knee Arthroplasty. *J. Arthroplast.* **2019**, *34*, 2347–2350. [CrossRef]
9. Setty, N.; LeBoff, M.S.; Thornhill, T.S.; Rinaldi, G.; Glowacki, J. Underestimated Fracture Probability in Patients With Unilateral Hip Osteoarthritis as Calculated by FRAX. *J. Clin. Densitom.* **2011**, *14*, 447–452. [CrossRef]
10. Puth, M.-T.; Klaschik, M.; Schmid, M.; Weckbecker, K.; Münster, E. Prevalence and Comorbidity of Osteoporosis—A Cross-Sectional Analysis on 10,660 Adults Aged 50 Years and Older in Germany. *BMC Musculoskelet. Disord.* **2018**, *19*, 144. [CrossRef]
11. Notarnicola, A.; Maccagnano, G.; Tafuri, S.; Moretti, L.; Laviola, L.; Moretti, B. Epidemiology of Diabetes Mellitus in the Fragility Fracture Population of a Region of Southern Italy. *J. Biol. Regul. Homeost. Agents* **2016**, *30*, 297–302. [PubMed]
12. Notarnicola, A.; Tafuri, S.; Maccagnano, G.; Moretti, L.; Moretti, B. Frequency of Hypertension in Hospitalized Population with Osteoporotic Fractures: Epidemiological Retrospective Analysis of Hospital Discharge Data in the Apulian Database for the Period 2006–2010. *Eur. J. Inflamm.* **2017**, *15*, 53–56. [CrossRef]
13. Ciatti, C.; Maniscalco, P.; Quattrini, F.; Gattoni, S.; Magro, A.; Capelli, P.; Banchini, F.; Fiazza, C.; Pavone, V.; Pagliarello, C.P.; et al. The Epidemiology of Proximal Femur Fractures during Covid-19 Emergency in Italy: A Multicentric Study. *Acta Biomed.* **2021**, *92*, e2021398. [CrossRef] [PubMed]
14. Dachverband Osteologie e.V. Prophylaxe, Diagnostik und Therapie der OSTEOPOROSE. Available online: https://www.dv-osteologie.org/uploads/Leitlinie2017/FinaleVersionLeitlinieOsteoporose2017_end.pdf (accessed on 1 January 2020).
15. Kanis, J.A.; Harvey, N.C.; McCloskey, E.; Bruyère, O.; Veronese, N.; Lorentzon, M.; Cooper, C.; Rizzoli, R.; Adib, G.; Al-Daghri, N.; et al. Algorithm for the Management of Patients at Low, High and Very High Risk of Osteoporotic Fractures. *Osteoporos. Int.* **2020**, *31*, 1–12. [CrossRef] [PubMed]

16. Neuerburg, C.; Mittlmeier, L.; Schmidmaier, R.; Kammerlander, C.; Böcker, W.; Mutschler, W.; Stumpf, U. Investigation and Management of Osteoporosis in Aged Trauma Patients: A Treatment Algorithm Adapted to the German Guidelines for Osteoporosis. *J. Orthop. Surg. Res.* **2017**, *12*, 86. [CrossRef] [PubMed]
17. Boudreau, D.M.; Yu, O.; Balasubramanian, A.; Wirtz, H.; Grauer, A.; Crittenden, D.B.; Scholes, D. A Survey of Women's Awareness of and Reasons for Lack of Postfracture Osteoporotic Care. *J. Am. Geriatr. Soc.* **2017**, *65*, 1829–1835. [CrossRef] [PubMed]
18. Ziller, V.; Kostev, K.; Kyvernitakis, I.; Boeckhoff, J.; Hadji, P. Persistence and Compliance of Medications Used in the Treatment of Osteoporosis—Analysis Using a Large Scale, Representative, Longitudinal German Database. *Int. J. Clin. Pharmacol. Ther.* **2012**, *50*, 315–322. [CrossRef]
19. Murad, M.H.; Drake, M.T.; Mullan, R.J.; Mauck, K.F.; Stuart, L.M.; Lane, M.A.; Abu Elnour, N.O.; Erwin, P.J.; Hazem, A.; Puhan, M.A.; et al. Comparative Effectiveness of Drug Treatments to Prevent Fragility Fractures: A Systematic Review and Network Meta-Analysis. *J. Clin. Endocrinol. Metab.* **2012**, *97*, 1871–1880. [CrossRef]
20. Karachalios, T.S.; Koutalos, A.A.; Komnos, G.A. Total Hip Arthroplasty in Patients with Osteoporosis. *HIP Int.* **2020**, *30*, 370–379. [CrossRef]
21. Russell, L.A. Osteoporosis and Orthopedic Surgery: Effect of Bone Health on Total Joint Arthroplasty Outcome. *Curr. Rheumatol. Rep.* **2013**, *15*, 371. [CrossRef]
22. Mundi, S.; Pindiprolu, B.; Simunovic, N.; Bhandari, M. Similar Mortality Rates in Hip Fracture Patients over the Past 31 Years. *Acta Orthop.* **2014**, *85*, 54–59. [CrossRef] [PubMed]
23. Lyles, K.W.; Colón-Emeric, C.S.; Magaziner, J.S.; Adachi, J.D.; Pieper, C.F.; Mautalen, C.; Hyldstrup, L.; Recknor, C.; Nordsletten, L.; Moore, K.A.; et al. Zoledronic Acid and Clinical Fractures and Mortality after Hip Fracture. *N. Engl. J. Med.* **2007**, *357*, 1799–1809. [CrossRef] [PubMed]
24. Åkesson, K.E.; McGuigan, F.E.A. Closing the Osteoporosis Care Gap. *Curr. Osteoporos. Rep.* **2021**, *19*, 58–65. [CrossRef] [PubMed]
25. Gosch, M.; Kammerlander, C.; Neuerburg, C. Osteoporosis—Epidemiology and Quality of Care. *Z. Gerontol. Geriatr.* **2019**, *52*, 408–413. [CrossRef] [PubMed]
26. Geiger, I.; Kammerlander, C.; Höfer, C.; Volland, R.; Trinemeier, J.; Henschelchen, M.; Friess, T.; FLS-CARE study group; Böcker, W.; Sundmacher, L. Implementation of an Integrated Care Programme to Avoid Fragility Fractures of the Hip in Older Adults in 18 Bavarian Hospitals—Study Protocol for the Cluster-Randomised Controlled Fracture Liaison Service FLS-CARE. *BMC Geriatr.* **2021**, *21*, 43. [CrossRef] [PubMed]

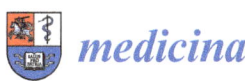

Review

Proximal Femoral Fractures in the Elderly: A Few Things to Know, and Some to Forget

Nicola Maffulli [1,2,3,4,*] and Rocco Aicale [1,2]

1. Department of Musculoskeletal Disorders, Faculty of Medicine and Surgery, University of Salerno, 84084 Baronissi, Italy
2. Clinica Ortopedica, Ospedale San Giovanni di Dio e Ruggi D'Aragona, 84131 Salerno, Italy
3. Barts and the London School of Medicine and Dentistry, Queen Mary University of London, Centre for Sports and Exercise Medicine, Mile End Hospital, London E1 4DG, UK
4. School of Pharmacology and Bioengineering, Guy Hilton Research Centre, Faculty of Medicine, Keele University, Thornburrow Drive, Hartshill, Stoke-on-Trent ST4 7QB, UK
* Correspondence: n.maffulli@qmul.ac.uk; Tel.: +44-20-8567-7553

Abstract: Hip fractures are a leading cause of hospitalisation in elderly patients, representing an increasing socioeconomic problem arising from demographic changes, considering the increased number of elderly people in our countries. Adequate peri-operative treatment is essential to decrease mortality rates and avoid complications. Modern management should involve a coordinated multidisciplinary approach, early surgery, pain treatment, balanced fluid therapy, and prevention of delirium, to improve patients' functional and clinical outcomes. The operative treatment for intertrochanteric and subtrochanteric fractures is intramedullary nail or sliding/dynamic hip screw (DHS) on the basis of the morphology of the fracture. In the case of neck fractures, total hip replacement (THR) or hemiarthroplasty are recommended. However, several topics remain debated, such as the optimum thromboprophylaxis to reduce venous thromboembolism or the use of bone cement. Postoperatively, patients can benefit from early mobilisation and geriatric multidisciplinary care. However, during the COVID-19 pandemic, a prolonged time to operation with a subsequent increased complication rate have burdened frail and elderly patients with hip fractures. Future studies are needed with the aim to investigate better strategies to improve nutrition, postoperative mobility, to clarify the role of home-based rehabilitation, and to identify the ideal analgesic treatment and adequate tools in case of patients with cognitive impairment.

Keywords: elderly; nailing; hip; proximal hip fracture; COVID-19

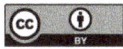

1. Introduction

Proximal femur fractures are a common consequence of osteoporosis, and we refer collectively to them as "hip fractures". They are a global challenge for healthcare systems and for patients themselves and their families, as there were 1.31 million of hip fractures in 1990 [1], and they are predicted to rise to 6.26 million globally by 2050 [2,3]. The socioeconomic costs represent 0.1% of the global burden of disease worldwide [1]. Hip fractures are potentially a catastrophic event: about 30% of such patients will die within the first year after injury [4], and the survivors will experience an increasing ongoing burden of illness which will affect their quality of life [5]. Within 1 year following the fracture, only between 40 and 60% of such elderly patients will have returned to their pre-injury level of mobility and ability [6].

Several evidence-based guidelines are supported by systematic reviews, and such patients commonly present the association of different metabolic (diabetic and thyroid disease) and inflammatory diseases [7–11].

Patients older than 80 or patients with common elderly multimorbidity aged over 70 are defined as "geriatric" [12], and 25 to 50% of patients over 85 are considered frail [13].

Frailty is a specific condition described as an increased vulnerability to stressors [13], and frailty fractures are defined as bone damage in the absence of important trauma or following a fall from standing height or less; in this context, hip fractures are the most common type of frailty fracture [14,15].

Surgical management should take place within the first 24 h, beyond which there is an increased chance of peri-operative complications (i.e., pulmonary embolism, pneumonia, deep vein thrombosis (DVT), urinary tract infections). In case of surgery delay for more than 48 h, mortality may rise significantly [16]; however, if surgery is undertaken within 48 h, a 20% lower risk of dying during the next year has been reported [17].

During the COVID-19 global pandemic, the total number of hip fracture patients was significantly reduced [18]. However, a systematic review and meta-analysis have shown a seven-fold increased mortality risk for COVID-19-positive patients with hip fractures and an increase in postoperative complications [19]. The time necessary to obtain the results of COVID-19 tests, the reduced operating capacity, and the shortage of hospital staff were identified as the major challenges. A recent multicentre study showed a mean delay of 2.4 days to surgery, with a minimum of 0 days and a maximum of 13 days [20].

The identification and treatment of geriatric conditions and prevention of complications is the aim of a comprehensive geriatric assessment [7], and modern "hip fracture care" is a multidisciplinary effort which acknowledges that a hip fracture is not a simple fracture but a marker of general health status deterioration.

2. Diagnosis

Typically, proximal femoral fractures occur in the elderly as a result of low energy trauma (i.e., a fall from standing). In the UK, the last report of the National Hip Fracture database (NHFD) reveals that 91.6% of hip fractures occur in patients over 70, and 72% are females [21], reflecting the increasing probability of falling (in the over 65 years, one in three people fall each year) and osteoporosis with advancing age [22].

On examination, patients report hip pain and inability to bear weight, with the affected leg shortened and externally rotated. Plain radiographs are adequate for diagnosis, but, when they are apparently normal with clinical signs and symptoms suggestive of a hip fracture, magnetic resonance imaging (MRI) or computed tomography (CT) may be indicated, i.e., the so-called "occult hip fracture", [23].

3. Classification

Hip fractures can be divided into intra and extracapsular, respectively, inside or outside the hip joint capsule, reflecting the disrupted blood supply of the femoral head, and guiding the decision process as to whether the patient will undergo (hemi) arthroplasty or internal fixation of intra-capsular fractures, and the choice of which construct to use to stabilise extracapsular fractures (i.e., intramedullary fixation with a nail or extramedullary fixation with a sliding hip screw) (Figure 1) [2,24].

Generally, patients will undergo surgery, obtaining benefits of the early fixation/replacement such as rapid postoperative mobilisation, and avoiding the poor outcomes and risks associated with long-term immobilisation from nonoperative treatment [25].

Intracapsular fractures are commonly divided in subcapital, midcervical, and basicervical; especially in the elderly, midcervical are the most common type, at over 86% of intracapsular fractures [26].

Three classifications for femoral neck fractures are the most common used: Garden's, Pauwels's (Figures 2 and 3), and the AO classification.

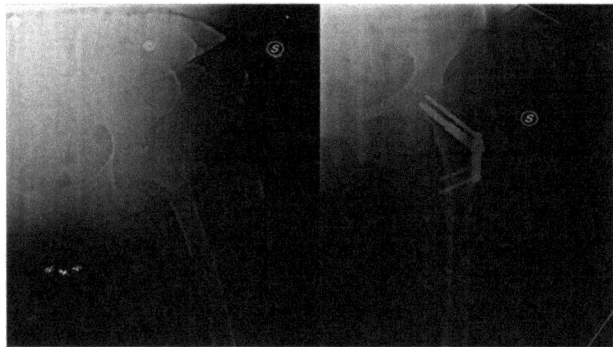

Figure 1. Dynamic hip screw (DHS), pre and post operation of hip fracture using a particular type of DHS, named Anteversa Plate.

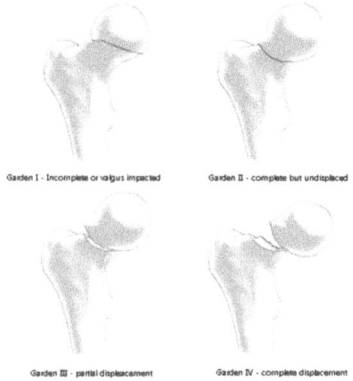

Figure 2. Garden classification.

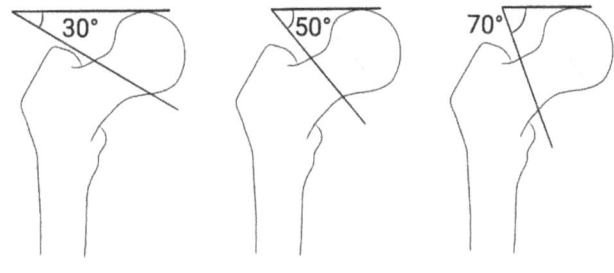

Figure 3. Pauwels classification.

The Garden classification, characterised by a fair inter-observer reliability, is composed of four types: type I describes an incomplete or impacted fracture; type II a complete fracture without displacement; type III a complete fracture with partial displacement; and type IV a complete fracture with full displacement [27].

The Pauwels classification is based on biomechanical forces and pressure at the fracture line site: in type I, a compression force is dominating, with a fracture line up to 30° to the horizontal plane; in type II there is a shearing stress, with negative impact on bone healing [28] and with a fracture line between 30° and 50°; in type III, the fracture line is above 50° with shearing stress being the predominant force, leading to fracture displacement [29]. However, for this classification, a weak reliability and reproducibility have been reported [30].

Probably, the most complete classification is the AO classification which combines the fracture level, degree of displacement, and fracture line angle. The original version of the (AO)/ASIF classification for hip fracture has been in use since 1990 [31], and it has rapidly become popular and readily used in the scientific literature. The new AO/OTA classification, published in 2018, imparts greater importance to the integrity of the lateral wall, which may play an important role in decision making and has been identified as a major prognostic factor to predict mechanical failure after surgery [32]. Furthermore, the AO/OTA classification considers isolated trochanteric fractures (of the greater or lesser trochanter), which were not classified in the original AO system.

4. Peri-Operative Pharmacological Management

Pain management is mandatory given its essential role in delirium prevention [33]. However, in the elderly, NSAIDs are not recommended, and drugs such as paracetamol every 6 h, unless contraindicated, can be useful [34]. When pain control is not achieved, oral opioids can be administered and accompanied by constipation prophylaxis [16].

Routine laboratory tests should include complete blood count, inflammation markers, prothrombin time—international normalised ratio (PT-INR), partial thromboplastin time, and metabolic profile [16]. Given their age, frequently, patients with hip fractures tend to be dehydrated; a flow rate of 100–200 mL/h of isotonic crystalloids is estimated to be safe [16].

The incidence of urinary tract infections and asymptomatic bacteriuria increases with age [35], and an association with superficial wound infections and symptomatic bacteriuria has been reported. A recent systematic literature review has shown that the postoperative infectious rate did not decrease if asymptomatic bacteriuria was treated before surgery [36]. Therefore, screening of the urinary tract infections is recommended, but treatment is needed only when symptomatic [16].

Thromboprophylaxis received great attention for hip fracture patients in the last few years given the risk of deep vein thrombosis (DVT), but the role of early surgery and mobilisation in mitigating this risk is clear.

Given the potential increase in morbidity and mortality from thromboembolic events, several national guidelines recommend thromboprophylaxis [8] and, at present, some evidence can be found supporting the graduated compression stockings and cyclical leg compression devices to reduce DVT with relatively good compliance and little risk of skin abrasions [37,38].

Regarding bleeding complications prevention, 40% of elderly patients with hip fractures take anticoagulants or antiplatelet agents [39], and optimal coordination with anaesthesiologists is mandatory: in patients with antiplatelet therapy, the recommendation is to proceed with the surgery with no delay [40]. In the case of double antiplatelet therapy, spinal anaesthesia is contraindicated [40]. Furthermore, a PT-INR value below 1.5 is an indication for vitamin K antagonists, including warfarin and phenprocoumon [40].

The use of clopidogrel and aspirin can increase perioperative blood loss, but hip fracture surgery can still safely be performed with no delay [41].

In patients with mechanical valves, atrial fibrillation (AF), with recent stroke history, DVT, or pulmonary embolism, the use of subcutaneous low-molecular weight heparin or intravenous unfractionated heparin need to be taken into consideration [42].

In the case of patients who use anti-Xa-agents (Apixaban, Edoxaban, Rivaroxaban), a plasma drug level of under 50 pg/mL is deemed safe for surgery, and, if the plasma level cannot be measured, a 24 h gap between the last dose and surgery should be considered [43].

Systemic tranexamic acid administration reduces blood loss and transfusion rates, impacting favourably on post-operative bleeding and not interfering with anti-coagulation. However, a recent meta-analysis could not ascertain what its optimal regimen, timing, and dosage are [44].

Delirium can be present, and often it remains undiagnosed in the elderly [45], increasing complications and mortality risks. Its prevention can play an essential role in the care of hip fracture patients [46]. Screening for delirium is not simple, but questionnaires such as the 4AT, a sensitive and specific tool, are validated for hip fractures [47], and can be used to evaluate mental status changes. They should be used in routine screening on admission. Multicomponent non-pharmacological approaches have been used, showing good results and including early mobilisation, adequate hydration, sleep enhancement, orientation in time and place, and therapeutic activities such as reminiscence [45]. An ideal policy for visitors can be adjusted to achieve a reduction in stress and maintain routine activities and a normal night–day rhythm.

5. Surgical Management

Hip fractures are an emergency, and strong evidence regarding early surgery is associated with a reduction in the risk of death [48].

Treatment should aim to return patients to their previous levels of daily life activities and full weight bearing. Management depends on the different type of hip fracture, based on the vascular anatomy of the proximal femur and the different chances of bone healing and future complications.

Regarding intertrochanteric and subtrochanteric fractures, surgical management is intramedullary nailing, which allows the decrease in soft tissue injuries during surgery and early weight-bearing after surgery (Figure 4). The implant choice for intertrochanteric fractures depends on fracture stability defined by the lateral cortical wall [49]. For example, extramedullary devices such as the sliding hip screw (SHS) can be chosen when the lateral cortex is intact, but an intramedullary device has biomechanical advantages given its location closer to the vector of the force of gravity, due to a shorter lever arm compared to extramedullary devices [24,49].

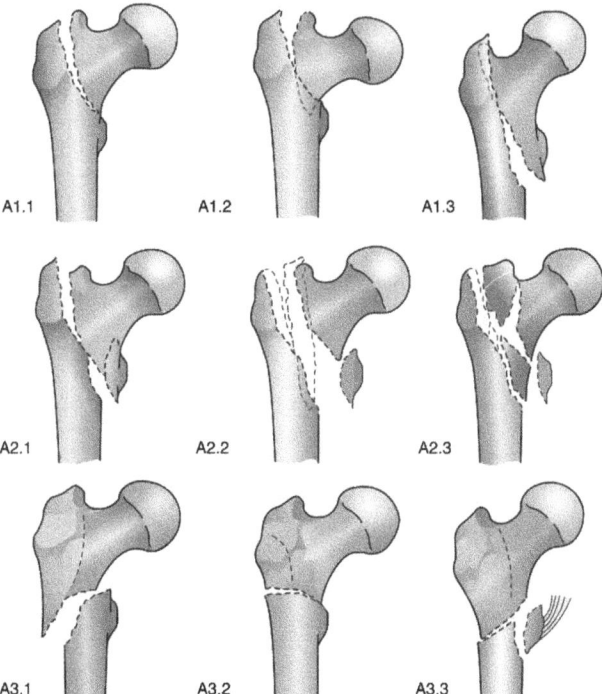

Figure 4. AO/OTA classification and subclassification.

A recent meta-analysis comparing different management options for intertrochanteric fractures [dynamic hip screw, compression hip screw, percutaneous compression plate, Medoff sliding plate, less invasive stabilisation system, gamma nail, proximal femoral nail, and proximal femoral nail anti-rotating (PFNA)] identified the PFNA as the option with less blood loss and higher functional results [50].

The use of the helical blade in intramedullary devices resulted in a higher collapse rate of the neck-shaft angle with a cut-out of the screw compared to the lag screw [51].

A recent prospective randomised controlled trial in hip fracture patients showed that the use of nail and cephalic hydroxyapatite coated screws results in higher mechanical stability and improved implant osteointegration compared to standard nailing [52].

A less common type of hip fracture is the subtrochanteric fracture, for which intramedullary nailing with a long nail is the accepted standard, given the reduced operation time, fixation failure rate, and length of stay (LOS) when compared to extramedullary devices [53].

SHSs are an established and optimal option to manage extra-capsular hip fractures, in particular the extra-capsular AO/OTA A1 and A2 fractures avoiding fracture collapse with good mechanical stability [54,55]. However, in the case of more complex unstable fractures (A3 types) with comminution and/or deficient bone to share the load with the fixation device, the fracture may collapse into varus with the consequent cut-out of the cephalic screw, or the femoral shaft may medialise excessively producing mechanical failure (Figure 5). An intramedullary nail for subtrochanteric fractures, and these types of fractures, achieves a more stable construct [56].

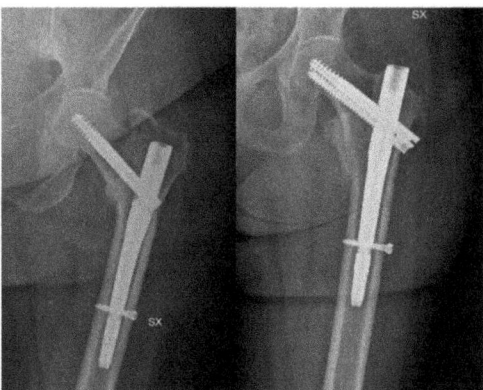

Figure 5. Hip fracture nailing using two different devices characterised by one or two cephalic screws

Despite the clear guidelines about the use of modern implants in certain fracture patterns, there still remain some gaps in the evidence [57].

Cement augmentation improves the stability of the implant in osteoporotic bone, but it has been linked to the risk of thermal damage, osteonecrosis, and cement leaking at the fracture site [58]. A recent systematic review on the clinical results of cement augmentation showed improved radiographic parameters and lower complication rates, but more studies are needed [59].

Femoral neck fractures can be managed conservatively or with surgery, using total hip arthroplasty (THA) or hemiarthroplasty. In the case of non-surgical treatment, patients with more than one comorbidity aged above 70 have an 83% risk of secondary dislocations of the fracture [60], making surgery the best choice in elderly patients. Displaced intra-capsular fractures are approximately half of all hip fractures [21], and they occur in a region where the femoral blood supply is tenuous, and healing is unreliable. Hip hemiarthroplasty, in which only the femoral head is replaced, is the treatment of choice, and current evidence supports the use of bone cement [61] (Figure 6).

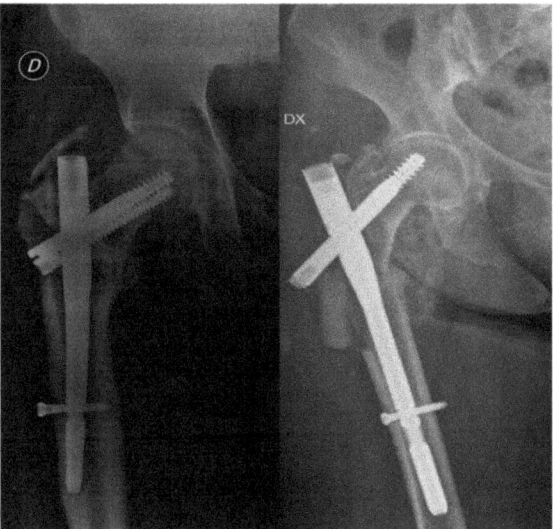

Figure 6. Failure examples of hip fracture fixation using nail devices.

For the choice of the implant, two main aspects need to be considered: indication for osteosynthesis, and, furthermore, consideration that elderly patients are less compliant to weight-bearing restrictions [62].

Following the Pauwels classification, in type I or II of femoral fractures, internal fixation is indicated. Considering femoral head blood supply, in type III and IV of the Garden classification fracture osteosynthesis is generally not recommended.

Displaced femoral neck fractures are generally accompanied by the disrupted blood supply predisposing to fixation failure; when there are co-existing osteoporosis and age-related bone changes, there is a major increase in the risk of non-unions in the elderly [63].

Osteosynthesis can be suggested as a salvage option or in young patients with non-placed fractures (Figure 7). If patients are bed-bound, surgery is indicated for pain management.

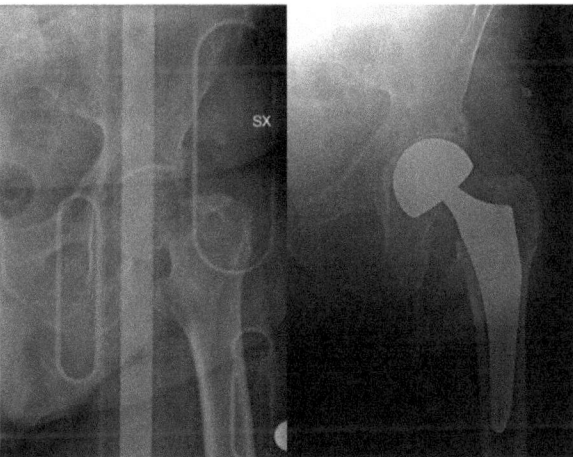

Figure 7. Treatment of fracture of neck of the femur using a hemiarthroplasty.

In the case of healthy and active patients, biological age can guide the implant choice: in the case of high functional requirements and lower biological age, indications shift towards THA instead of hemiarthroplasty, which is indicated in the healthy elderly [64] (Figure 8).

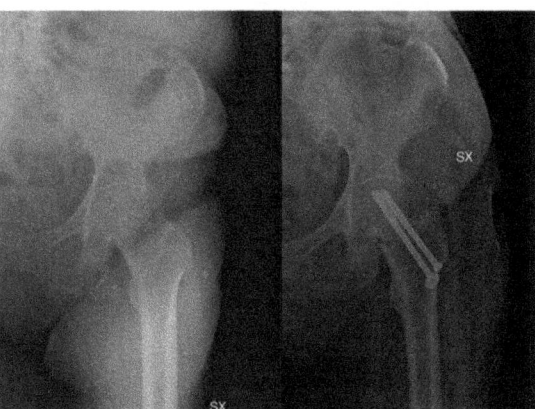

Figure 8. In young patients with non-displaced fractures or as a salvage option, two or three partially threaded canulated screws can be used.

Cemented implants are characterised by less postoperative pain and better mobility [61], with better fixation in the osteoporotic bone [65]. However, bone cement has risks, especially in frail patients, with an increased morbidity and mortality in intra and post-operative periods [66]. However, bone cement implantation syndrome is rare, and evidence highlights the reduction in pain and increased functional outcomes compared to uncemented implants [61].

The periprosthetic femoral fracture risk is two times higher in patients above 60 years with uncemented stems compared to cemented stems [67]. For those with an elevated risk and suitable bone quality, to reduce the risks of cement implantation syndrome during surgery, a non-cemented femoral component is indicated.

Cemented THA should be considered for patients with high levels of pre-injury activity and able to walk independently, with no cognitive impairment and medically fit to undergo a longer operation [57].

THA can be associated with a higher dislocation rate [65], but, in young and active patients, it remains the implant of choice given the optimal outcomes and lower long-term reoperation rate compared to hemiarthroplasty. The risk of dislocation is related to the components' positioning, surgeon's experience, and soft tissue tension, [68]. In elderly patients, sarcopenia, proprioception loss, and increased risk of falls are other factors which need to be considered [68] (Figure 9).

Hemiarthroplasty does have some advantages, such as shorter surgery time and lower dislocation incidence [64], but, in young patients, hemiarthroplasty has a high rate of acetabular erosion with the need for conversion in THA for secondary osteoarthritis [69].

A multicentre randomised controlled trial compared displaced femoral neck fractures managed either with THA or hemiarthroplasty, with no difference incidence of secondary interventions, but the better WOMAC score favoured THA over hemiarthroplasty [70].

Basicervical femoral neck fractures are uncommon (1.8% of cases), and management includes both a cephalomedullary nail and DHS. Cancellous screws are not recommended given their high failure rate. Further research with well-defined management outcomes or fixation failure evaluation are needed to achieve clear recommendations [71].

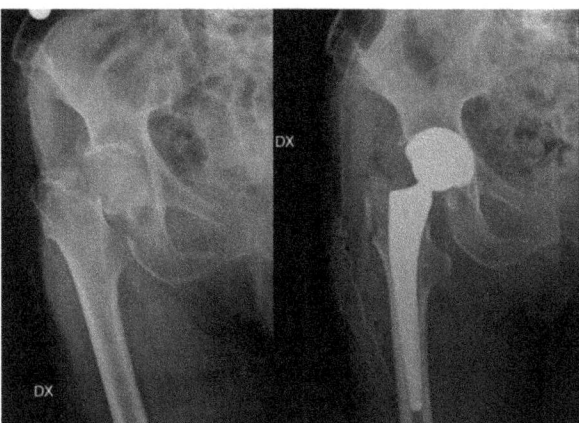

Figure 9. In case of healthy and active patients, with high functional requirements and lower biological age, total hip arthroplasty is the treatment of choice.

6. Postoperative Treatment

To reduce the risk of pneumonia, pressure ulcers, thromboembolism, and delirium, early mobilisation is recommended, particularly in elderly patients [72]. In general, patients who have had one fracture are at risk of another one, and for this reason it is essential to investigate the cause of the fractures and prevent further accidents, taking in consideration that syncope, Parkinson's disease, and polypharmacy are associated with an increased risk of falling in the elderly [73].

Postoperative care needs to include mechanical thromboembolism prophylaxis mediated by early mobilisation, pharmacological prophylaxis with low molecular-weight heparin continued for 28–35 days, and physiotherapy [74].

7. Postoperative Care

Fracture prevention plays an essential role for elderly care, and two strategies are employed: reduce fall risk and improve patients' overall bone health. To avoid the risk of falls, a clinical assessment to identify medical conditions (such as postural hypotension, syncope, arrhythmia) needs to be undertaken, and basic investigations (i.e., blood pressure measurements, a 12-lead ECG, and a review of current medications) can be helpful. Mechanical causes such as poor mobility and impaired vision need to be evaluated and managed, and a home assessment with relative modifications is recommended.

Bone health status can be obtained by routine blood tests to evaluate calcium or vitamin D deficiency, and a review of drugs used and comorbidities such as liver and renal disease. Secondary prevention of osteoporotic fracture is recommended in elderly patients with confirmed osteoporosis and high risk of re-fracture, with the initial use of anabolic drugs (such as teriparatide, abaloparatide, romosozumab) followed by anticatabolic drugs (i.e., oral or intravenous bisphosphonates or denosumab) [75].

The rehabilitation process begins with the involvement of specialists such as orthogeriatricians, who play a clear role to optimise the patient's medical condition in the perioperative period and early supported discharge [39,76]. Mobilisation is recommended already the day after surgery [77], and early intensive rehabilitation is more effective to improve mobility compared to a more sedate approach [78,79].

However, there is no consensus regarding which is the optimal strategy to improve mobility [80]. Only some high-quality studies investigate nutrition's role [81,82], and moderate evidence [83] supports dietary supplementation, to avoid protein and energy malnutrition, improving postoperative nutritional status and decreasing mortality [81].

8. Conclusions

Hip fractures are demanding challenges for patients and healthcare systems. Management cannot be limited to the operating theatre. Given the increase in the burden of disease, the true challenge is in prevention and in developing strategies to improve the quality of life for this group of patients.

Generally, an interdisciplinary orthogeriatric treatment reduces the length of hospital stay, number of complications, and mortality. Essential peri-operative aspects are pain management, early mobilisation, management of fluid, and delirium prevention.

The COVID-19 pandemic has brought additional difficulties in hip fracture patients' care, leading to a delay in surgery, and a higher complication rate. Despite the importance of this condition and its impact on the life quality of patients, our knowledge is still evolving and there remains a lack of quality evidence for management options that we can offer.

Author Contributions: One medical doctor (R.A.) performed articles search in the available scientific literature, while the researcher with more experience (N.M.) solved cases of doubt. At the beginning of the procedure, examiner read the abstracts of all articles, and selected the relevant ones. Each author has contributed to write the manuscript. All authors have read and agreed to the published version of the manuscript.

Funding: This research received no external funding.

Institutional Review Board Statement: Not applicable.

Informed Consent Statement: Not applicable.

Data Availability Statement: Not applicable.

Conflicts of Interest: The authors declare no conflict of interest.

References

1. Johnell, O.; Kanis, J.A. An estimate of the worldwide prevalence, mortality and disability associated with hip fracture. *Osteoporos. Int.* **2004**, *15*, 897–902. [CrossRef] [PubMed]
2. Aicale, R.; Maffulli, N. Greater rate of cephalic screw mobilisation following proximal femoral nailing in hip fractures with a tip-apex distance (TAD) and a calcar referenced TAD greater than 25 mm. *J. Orthop. Surg. Res.* **2018**, *13*, 106. [CrossRef] [PubMed]
3. Cooper, C.; Campion, G.; Melton, L.J. Hip fractures in the elderly: A world-wide projection. *Osteoporos. Int.* **1992**, *2*, 285–289. [CrossRef] [PubMed]
4. Roberts, S.E.; Goldacre, M.J. Time trends and demography of mortality after fractured neck of femur in an English population, 1968–1998: Database study. *BMJ* **2003**, *327*, 771–775. [CrossRef]
5. Griffin, X.L.; Parsons, N.; Achten, J.; Fernandez, M.; Costa, M.L. Recovery of health-related quality of life in a United Kingdom hip fracture population. The Warwick Hip Trauma Evaluation—A prospective cohort study. *Bone Jt. J.* **2015**, *97-B*, 372–382. [CrossRef]
6. Dyer, S.M.; Crotty, M.; Fairhall, N.; Magaziner, J.; Beaupre, L.A.; Cameron, I.D.; Sherrington, C.; Fragility Fracture Network (FFN) Rehabilitation Research Special Interest Group. A critical review of the long-term disability outcomes following hip fracture. *BMC Geriatr.* **2016**, *16*, 158. [CrossRef]
7. Aletto, C.; Aicale, R.; Pezzuti, G.; Bruno, F.; Maffulli, N. Impact of an orthogeriatrician on length of stay of elderly patient with hip fracture. *Osteoporos. Int.* **2020**, *31*, 2161–2166. [CrossRef]
8. Network SIG. Management of Hip Fracture in Older People: A National Clinical Guideline. 2009; Edinburgh: [cit 2018-04-05]. Available online: http://www.sign.ac.uk/assets/sign111.pdf (accessed on 2 August 2018).
9. Chehade, M.; Taylor, A. *Australian and New Zealand Guideline for Hip Fracture Care-Improving Outcomes in Hip Fracture Management of Adults*; Australian and New Zealand Hip Fracture Registry (ANZHFR): Randwick, Australia, 2014.
10. Maccagnano, G.; Notarnicola, A.; Pesce, V.; Mudoni, S.; Tafuri, S.; Moretti, B. The Prevalence of Fragility Fractures in a Population of a Region of Southern Italy Affected by Thyroid Disorders. *BioMed Res. Int.* **2016**, *2016*, 6017165. [CrossRef]
11. Notarnicola, A.; Maccagnano, G.; Tafuri, S.; Moretti, L.; Laviola, L.; Moretti, B. Epidemiology of diabetes mellitus in the fragility fracture population of a region of Southern Italy. *J. Biol. Regul. Homeost. Agents* **2016**, *30*, 297–302.
12. Sieber, C.C. Der ältere Patient—Wer ist das? *Der Internist* **2007**, *48*, 1190–1194. [CrossRef]
13. Clegg, A.; Young, J.; Iliffe, S.; Rikkert, M.O.; Rockwood, K. Frailty in elderly people. *Lancet* **2013**, *381*, 752–762. [CrossRef]
14. Harvey, N.C.W.; McCloskey, E.V.; Mitchell, P.J.; Dawson-Hughes, B.; Pierroz, D.D.; Reginster, J.-Y.; Rizzoli, R.; Cooper, C.; Kanis, J.A. Mind the (treatment) gap: A global perspective on current and future strategies for prevention of fragility fractures. *Osteoporos. Int.* **2017**, *28*, 1507–1529. [CrossRef]
15. Migliorini, F.; Giorgino, R.; Hildebrand, F.; Spiezia, F.; Peretti, G.M.; Alessandri-Bonetti, M.; Eschweiler, J.; Maffulli, N. Fragility Fractures: Risk Factors and Management in the Elderly. *Medicina* **2021**, *57*, 1119. [CrossRef]

16. Mears, S.C.; Kates, S.L. A Guide to Improving the Care of Patients with Fragility Fractures, Edition 2. *Geriatr. Orthop. Surg. Rehabil.* **2015**, *6*, 58–120. [CrossRef]
17. Klestil, T.; Röder, C.; Stotter, C.; Winkler, B.; Nehrer, S.; Lutz, M.; Klerings, I.; Wagner, G.; Gartlehner, G.; Nussbaumer-Streit, B. Impact of timing of surgery in elderly hip fracture patients: A systematic review and meta-analysis. *Sci. Rep.* **2018**, *8*, 13933. [CrossRef]
18. Kumar Jain, V.; Lal, H.; Kumar Patralekh, M.; Vaishya, R. Fracture management during COVID-19 pandemic: A systematic review. *J. Clin. Orthop. Trauma* **2020**, *11*, S431–S441. [CrossRef]
19. Lim, M.A.; Pranata, R. Coronavirus disease 2019 (COVID-19) markedly increased mortality in patients with hip fracture—A systematic review and meta-analysis. *J. Clin. Orthop. Trauma* **2021**, *12*, 187–193. [CrossRef]
20. Muñoz Vives, J.M.; Jornet-Gibert, M.; Cámara-Cabrera, J.; Esteban, P.L.; Brunet, L.; Delgado-Flores, L.; Camacho-Carrasco, P.; Torner, P.; Marcano-Fernández, F.; Spanish HIP-COVID Investigation Group. Mortality Rates of Patients with Proximal Femoral Fracture in a Worldwide Pandemic: Preliminary Results of the Spanish HIP-COVID Observational Study. *J. Bone Jt. Surg. Am.* **2020**, *102*, e69. [CrossRef]
21. Royal College of Physicians. *Falls and Fragility Fracture Audit Programme*; Physiotherapy 'Hip Sprint' Audit Report London; Royal College of Physicians: London, UK, 2017.
22. De Laet, C.E.; Pols, H.A. Fractures in the elderly: Epidemiology and demography. *Best Pract. Res. Clin. Endocrinol. Metab.* **2000**, *14*, 171–179. [CrossRef]
23. Chatha, H.A.; Ullah, S.; Cheema, Z.Z. Review article: Magnetic resonance imaging and computed tomography in the diagnosis of occult proximal femur fractures. *J. Orthop. Surg.* **2011**, *19*, 99–103. [CrossRef]
24. Aicale, R.; Tarantino, D.; Oliviero, G.; Maccauro, G.; Peretti, G.M.; Maffulli, N. O'nil Anteversa® mini-plate for stable hip fracture: First experience considerations and outcomes. *J. Biol. Regul. Homeost. Agents* **2019**, *33*, 147–154. [PubMed]
25. Gillespie, W.J. Extracts from "clinical evidence": Hip fracture. *BMJ* **2001**, *322*, 968–975. [CrossRef] [PubMed]
26. Beck, A.; Rüter, A. Schenkelhalsfrakturen-Diagnostik und therapeutisches Vorgehen. *Der Unfallchirurg* **1998**, *101*, 634–648. [CrossRef] [PubMed]
27. Garden, R.S. Low-angle fixation in fractures of the femoral neck. *J. Bone Jt. Surg. Br. Vol.* **1961**, *43*, 647–663. [CrossRef]
28. Steiner, M.; Claes, L.; Ignatius, A.; Simon, U.; Wehner, T. Disadvantages of interfragmentary shear on fracture healing—Mechanical insights through numerical simulation. *J. Orthop. Res.* **2014**, *32*, 865–872. [CrossRef]
29. Bartoníček, J. Pauwels' classification of femoral neck fractures: Correct interpretation of the original. *J. Orthop. Trauma* **2001**, *15*, 358–360. [CrossRef]
30. Gašpar, D.; Crnković, T.; Đurović, D.; Podsednik, D.; Slišurić, F. AO group, AO subgroup, Garden and Pauwels classification systems of femoral neck fractures: Are they reliable and reproducible? *Med. Glas.* **2012**, *9*, 243–247.
31. Meling, T.; Harboe, K.; Enoksen, C.H.; Aarflot, M. How reliable and accurate is the AO/OTA comprehensive classification for adult long-bone fractures? *J. Trauma Acute Care Surg.* **2012**, *73*, 224–231. [CrossRef]
32. Hsu, C.-E.; Huang, K.-C.; Lin, T.-C.; Tong, K.-M.; Lee, M.-H.; Chiu, Y.-C. Integrated risk scoring model for predicting dynamic hip screw treatment outcome of intertrochanteric fracture. *Injury* **2016**, *47*, 2501–2506. [CrossRef]
33. Eamer, G.; Taheri, A.; Chen, S.S.; Daviduck, Q.; Chambers, T.; Shi, X.; Khadaroo, R.G. Comprehensive geriatric assessment for older people admitted to a surgical service. *Cochrane Database Syst. Rev.* **2018**, *1*, CD012485. [CrossRef]
34. Ftouh, S.; Morga, A.; Swift, C. Management of hip fracture in adults: Summary of NICE guidance. *BMJ* **2011**, *342*, d3304. [CrossRef]
35. Rodriguez-Mañas, L. Urinary tract infections in the elderly: A review of disease characteristics and current treatment options. *Drugs Context* **2020**, *9*, 2020-4-13. [CrossRef]
36. Zhang, Q.; Liu, L.; Sun, W.; Gao, F.; Cheng, L.; Li, Z. Research progress of asymptomatic bacteriuria before arthroplasty: A systematic review. *Medicine* **2018**, *97*, e9810. [CrossRef]
37. Oliver, D.; Griffiths, R.; Roche, J.; Sahota, O. Hip fracture. *BMJ Clin. Evid.* **2010**, *2010*, 1110.
38. Handoll, H.H.; Farrar, M.J.; McBirnie, J.; Tytherleigh-Strong, G.; Milne, A.A.; Gillespie, W.J. Heparin, low molecular weight heparin and physical methods for preventing deep vein thrombosis and pulmonary embolism following surgery for hip fractures. *Cochrane Database Syst. Rev.* **2002**, *4*. [CrossRef]
39. Crotty, M.; Whitehead, C.H.; Gray, S.; Finucane, P.M. Early discharge and home rehabilitation after hip fracture achieves functional improvements: A randomized controlled trial. *Clin. Rehabil.* **2002**, *16*, 406–413. [CrossRef]
40. Yang, Z.; Ni, J.; Long, Z.; Kuang, L.; Gao, Y.; Tao, S. Is hip fracture surgery safe for patients on antiplatelet drugs and is it necessary to delay surgery? A systematic review and meta-analysis. *J. Orthop. Surg. Res.* **2020**, *15*, 105. [CrossRef]
41. Chechik, O.; Thein, R.; Fichman, G.; Haim, A.; Tov, T.B.; Steinberg, E.L. The effect of clopidogrel and aspirin on blood loss in hip fracture surgery. *Injury* **2011**, *42*, 1277–1282. [CrossRef]
42. Falaschi, P.; Marsh, D. (Eds.) *Orthogeriatrics: The Management of Older Patients with Fragility Fractures*; Springer: Cham, Switzerland, 2021.
43. Bonnaire, F.; Bula, P.; Schellong, S. Management vorbestehender Antikoagulation zur zeitgerechten Versorgung von hüftnahen Frakturen. *Der Unfallchirurg* **2019**, *122*, 404–410. [CrossRef]
44. Zhang, P.; He, J.; Fang, Y.; Chen, P.; Liang, Y.; Wang, J. Efficacy and safety of intravenous tranexamic acid administration in patients undergoing hip fracture surgery for hemostasis: A meta-analysis. *Medicine* **2017**, *96*, e6940. [CrossRef]

45. Oh, E.S.; Fong, T.G.; Hshieh, T.T.; Inouye, S.K. Delirium in Older Persons: Advances in Diagnosis and Treatment. *JAMA* **2017**, *318*, 1161–1174. [CrossRef]
46. Kim, S.-Y.; Kim, S.-W.; Kim, J.-M.; Shin, I.-S.; Bae, K.-Y.; Shim, H.-J.; Bae, W.-K.; Cho, S.-H.; Chung, I.-J.; Yoon, J.-S. Differential Associations Between Delirium and Mortality According to Delirium Subtype and Age: A Prospective Cohort Study. *Psychosom. Med.* **2015**, *77*, 903–910. [CrossRef]
47. Bellelli, G.; Morandi, A.; Davis, D.H.J.; Mazzola, P.; Turco, R.; Gentile, S.; Ryan, T.; Cash, H.; Guerini, F.; Torpilliesi, T.; et al. Validation of the 4AT, a new instrument for rapid delirium screening: A study in 234 hospitalised older people. *Age Ageing* **2014**, *43*, 496–502. [CrossRef] [PubMed]
48. Moja, L.; Piatti, A.; Pecoraro, V.; Ricci, C.; Virgili, G.; Salanti, G.; Germagnoli, L.; Liberati, A.; Banfi, G. Timing matters in hip fracture surgery: Patients operated within 48 hours have better outcomes. A meta-analysis and meta-regression of over 190,000 patients. *PLoS ONE* **2012**, *7*, e46175. [CrossRef]
49. Lu, Y.; Uppal, H.S. Hip Fractures: Relevant Anatomy, Classification, and Biomechanics of Fracture and Fixation. *Geriatr. Orthop. Surg. Rehabil.* **2019**, *10*, 2151459319859139. [CrossRef]
50. Yx, C.; Xia, S. Optimal surgical methods to treat intertrochanteric fracture: A Bayesian network meta-analysis based on 36 randomized controlled trials. *J. Orthop. Surg. Res.* **2020**, *15*, 402. [CrossRef]
51. Cipollaro, L.; Aicale, R.; Maccauro, G.; Maffulli, N. Single- versus double-integrated screws in intramedullary nailing systems for surgical management of extracapsular hip fractures in the elderly: A systematic review. *J. Biol. Regul. Homeost. Agents* **2019**, *33*, 175–182. [PubMed]
52. Pesce, V.; Maccagnano, G.; Vicenti, G.; Notarnicola, A.; Moretti, L.; Tafuri, S.; Vanni, D.; Salini, V.; Moretti, B. The effect of hydroxyapatite coated screw in the lateral fragility fractures of the femur. A prospective randomized clinical study. *J. Biol. Regul. Homeost. Agents* **2014**, *28*, 125–132. [PubMed]
53. Jackson, C.; Tanios, M.; Ebraheim, N. Management of Subtrochanteric Proximal Femur Fractures: A Review of Recent Literature. *Adv. Orthop.* **2018**, *2018*, 1326701. [CrossRef]
54. Queally, J.M.; Harris, E.; Handoll, H.H.G.; Parker, M.J. Intramedullary nails for extracapsular hip fractures in adults. *Cochrane Database Syst. Rev.* **2014**, *12*, CD004961. [CrossRef] [PubMed]
55. Parker, M.J.; Handoll, H.H. Gamma and other cephalocondylic intramedullary nails versus extramedullary implants for extracapsular hip fractures in adults. *Cochrane Database Syst. Rev.* **2010**, *8*, CD000093. [CrossRef]
56. Anglen, J.O.; Weinstein, J.N.; American Board of Orthopaedic Surgery Research Committee. Nail or plate fixation of intertrochanteric hip fractures: Changing pattern of practice: A review of the American Board of Orthopaedic Surgery Database. *J. Bone Jt. Surg. Am.* **2008**, *90*, 700–707. [CrossRef]
57. Chesser, T.J.S.; Handley, R.; Swift, C. New NICE guideline to improve outcomes for hip fracture patients. *Injury* **2011**, *42*, 727–729. [CrossRef]
58. Erhart, S.; Schmoelz, W.; Blauth, M.; Lenich, A. Biomechanical effect of bone cement augmentation on rotational stability and pull-out strength of the Proximal Femur Nail Antirotation™. *Injury* **2011**, *42*, 1322–1327. [CrossRef]
59. Namdari, S.; Rabinovich, R.; Scolaro, J.; Baldwin, K.; Bhandari, M.; Mehta, S. Absorbable and non-absorbable cement augmentation in fixation of intertrochanteric femur fractures: Systematic review of the literature. *Arch. Orthop. Trauma Surg.* **2013**, *133*, 487–494. [CrossRef]
60. Raaymakers, E.L.F.B. The non-operative treatment of impacted femoral neck fractures. *Injury* **2002**, *33* (Suppl. S3), C8–C14. [CrossRef]
61. Parker, M.J.; Gurusamy, K.S.; Azegami, S. Arthroplasties (with and without bone cement) for proximal femoral fractures in adults. *Cochrane Database Syst. Rev.* **2010**, *16*, CD001706. [CrossRef]
62. Kammerlander, C.; Pfeufer, D.; Lisitano, L.A.; Mehaffey, S.; Bocker, W.; Neuerburg, C. Inability of Older Adult Patients with Hip Fracture to Maintain Postoperative Weight-Bearing Restrictions. *J. Bone Jt. Surg. Am.* **2018**, *100*, 936–941. [CrossRef]
63. Lowe, J.A.; Crist, B.D.; Bhandari, M.; Ferguson, T.A. Optimal treatment of femoral neck fractures according to patient's physiologic age: An evidence-based review. *Orthop. Clin. N. Am.* **2010**, *41*, 157–166. [CrossRef]
64. Braun, K.F.; Hanschen, M.; Biberthaler, P. Frakturendoprothetik der medialen Schenkelhalsfraktur. *Der Unfallchirurg* **2016**, *119*, 331–345. [CrossRef]
65. Rozell, J.C.; Hasenauer, M.; Donegan, D.J.; Neuman, M. Recent advances in the treatment of hip fractures in the elderly. *F1000Res* **2016**, *5*, 1953. [CrossRef] [PubMed]
66. Rutter, P.D.; Panesar, S.S.; Darzi, A.; Donaldson, L.J. What is the risk of death or severe harm due to bone cement implantation syndrome among patients undergoing hip hemiarthroplasty for fractured neck of femur? A patient safety surveillance study. *BMJ Open* **2014**, *4*, e004853. [CrossRef] [PubMed]
67. Konow, T.; Baetz, J.; Melsheimer, O.; Grimberg, A.; Morlock, M. Factors influencing periprosthetic femoral fracture risk. *Bone Jt. J.* **2021**, *103-B*, 650–658. [CrossRef] [PubMed]
68. Dargel, J.; Oppermann, J.; Brüggemann, G.-P.; Eysel, P. Dislocation following total hip replacement. *Dtsch. Arztebl. Int.* **2014**, *111*, 884–890. [CrossRef]
69. Baker, R.P.; Squires, B.; Gargan, M.F.; Bannister, G.C. Total hip arthroplasty and hemiarthroplasty in mobile, independent patients with a displaced intracapsular fracture of the femoral neck. A randomized, controlled trial. *J. Bone Jt. Surg. Am.* **2006**, *88*, 2583–2589. [CrossRef]

70. Bhandari, M.; Einhorn, T.A.; Guyatt, G.; Schemitsch, E.H.; Zura, R.D.; Sprague, S.; Frihagen, F.; Guerra-Farfán, E.; Kleinlugtenbelt, Y.V.; Health Investigators. Total Hip Arthroplasty or Hemiarthroplasty for Hip Fracture. *N. Engl. J. Med.* **2019**, *381*, 2199–2208. [CrossRef]
71. Yoo, J.-I.; Cha, Y.; Kwak, J.; Kim, H.-Y.; Choy, W.-S. Review on Basicervical Femoral Neck Fracture: Definition, Treatments, and Failures. *Hip Pelvis* **2020**, *32*, 170–181. [CrossRef]
72. Kenyon-Smith, T.; Nguyen, E.; Oberai, T.; Jarsma, R. Early mobilization post–hip fracture surgery. *Geriatr. Orthop. Surg. Rehabil.* **2019**, *10*, 2151459319826431. [CrossRef]
73. Hammond, T.; Wilson, A. Polypharmacy and falls in the elderly: A literature review. *Nurs. Midwifery Stud.* **2013**, *2*, 171–175. [CrossRef]
74. Flevas, D.A.; Megaloikonomos, P.D.; Dimopoulos, L.; Mitsiokapa, E.; Koulouvaris, P.; Mavrogenis, A.F. Thromboembolism prophylaxis in orthopaedics: An update. *EFORT Open Rev.* **2018**, *3*, 136–148. [CrossRef]
75. Migliorini, F.; Colarossi, G.; Baroncini, A.; Eschweiler, J.; Tingart, M.; Maffulli, N. Pharmacological Management of Postmenopausal Osteoporosis: A Level I Evidence Based—Expert Opinion. *Expert Rev. Clin. Pharm.* **2021**, *14*, 105–119. [CrossRef]
76. Kuisma, R. A randomized, controlled comparison of home versus institutional rehabilitation of patients with hip fracture. *Clin. Rehabil.* **2002**, *16*, 553–561. [CrossRef]
77. Halbert, J.; Crotty, M.; Whitehead, C.; Cameron, I.; Kurrle, S.; Graham, S.; Handoll, H.; Finnegan, T.; Jones, T.; Foley, A.; et al. Multi-disciplinary rehabilitation after hip fracture is associated with improved outcome: A systematic review. *J. Rehabil. Med.* **2007**, *39*, 507–512. [CrossRef]
78. Mangione, K.K.; Craik, R.L.; Palombaro, K.M.; Tomlinson, S.S.; Hofmann, M.T. Home-based leg-strengthening exercise improves function 1 year after hip fracture: A randomized controlled study. *J. Am. Geriatr. Soc.* **2010**, *58*, 1911–1917. [CrossRef]
79. Sylliaas, H.; Brovold, T.; Wyller, T.B.; Bergland, A. Progressive strength training in older patients after hip fracture: A randomised controlled trial. *Age Ageing* **2011**, *40*, 221–227. [CrossRef]
80. Handoll, H.H.; Sherrington, C.; Mak, J.C. Interventions for improving mobility after hip fracture surgery in adults. *Cochrane Database Syst. Rev.* **2011**, *16*, CD001704. [CrossRef]
81. Duncan, D.G.; Beck, S.J.; Hood, K.; Johansen, A. Using dietetic assistants to improve the outcome of hip fracture: A randomised controlled trial of nutritional support in an acute trauma ward. *Age Ageing* **2006**, *35*, 148–153. [CrossRef]
82. Eneroth, M.; Olsson, U.-B.; Thorngren, K.-G. Nutritional supplementation decreases hip fracture-related complications. *Clin. Orthop. Relat. Res.* **2006**, *451*, 212–217. [CrossRef]
83. Roberts, K.C.; Brox, W.T.; Jevsevar, D.S.; Sevarino, K. Management of hip fractures in the elderly. *JAAOS J. Am. Acad. Orthop. Surg.* **2015**, *23*, 131–137. [CrossRef]

MDPI
St. Alban-Anlage 66
4052 Basel
Switzerland
www.mdpi.com

Medicina Editorial Office
E-mail: medicina@mdpi.com
www.mdpi.com/journal/medicina

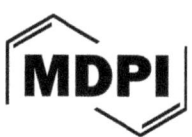

Disclaimer/Publisher's Note: The statements, opinions and data contained in all publications are solely those of the individual author(s) and contributor(s) and not of MDPI and/or the editor(s). MDPI and/or the editor(s) disclaim responsibility for any injury to people or property resulting from any ideas, methods, instructions or products referred to in the content.